The ACID REFLUX

COOKBOOK

101 Easy, Healthy & Fast Recipes to Relief from GERD and Avoid Any Worsening of Acid Reflux

28 DAY HELPFUL MEAL PLAN

ROBERT DICKENS & ANITA ROSE

Table of Contents

INTRODUCTION 9

THE BASICS OF ACID REFLUX 12

10 Important Things to Know if You Suffer From Acid Reflux 14

    Is it true that 8 glasses of water per day are good for you? 14

    Can sleep alleviate acid reflux? 16

    It is important to eat food at the right temperature 16

    Can recipes in this book help me treat my acid reflux? 17

    Complications Caused By Acid Reflux 17

    One particular thing about red meat in this diet that no one else will tell you 18

    You can eat legumes, but pay attention to one thing… 18

    Acid Reflux Can Be Linked to Diet 19

    Treatment Can Vary 19

    Losing Lots of Weight Is Not Necessary 19

At Home, Natural Remedies 20

FAQ 21

    Does Everyone Who Has Acid Reflux Have GERD? 21

    Can Children Develop GERD? 21

    Is There a Cure for GERD? 21

    Who Has a High Risk of Developing GERD? 21

Eating for Acid Reflux 22

    What to Eat 23

    What to Avoid 24

    What to Drink 25

    Food Swaps 26

    Food List 30

Meal Plan and Shopping List 32

    Building a Shopping List 32

    28 Day Meal Plan 33

RECIPES 43

MEASUREMENT CONVERSIONS 44

Breakfast 47

Banana Walnut Muffins	VEGETARIAN	48
Buttermilk Pancakes	VEGETARIAN	49
Granola	VEGETARIAN	50
Hash Browns	VEGAN	51
Overnight Oats	VEGETARIAN	52
Blueberry Muffins	VEGETARIAN	53
French Toast	VEGETARIAN	54
Roasted Vegetable Breakfast Tacos	VEGAN	55
Sweet Potato Toast With Ginger-Honey…	GLUTEN-FREE VEGAN	56
Simple Granola	VEGAN	57
Baked Apple Pancake	VEGETARIAN	58
Roasted Veggie and Goat Cheese Frittata	VEGETARIAN	59
Zucchini Bread	VEGETARIAN	60
Apple and Cinnamon Bread	VEGETARIAN	62

Smoothie 65

Sweet Pea Smoothie	GLUTEN-FREE VEGAN	66
Strawberry Banana Smoothie	GLUTEN-FREE VEGETARIAN	67
Tropical Melon Smoothie	GLUTEN-FREE VEGETARIAN	68
Green Smoothie	GLUTEN-FREE VEGAN	69
Kale and Ginger Smoothie	GLUTEN-FREE VEGAN	70
Spinach, Mango, and Melon Smoothie	GLUTEN-FREE VEGAN	71
Alkaline Smoothie	GLUTEN-FREE VEGAN	72
Melon Smoothie	GLUTEN-FREE VEGAN	73
Apple Smoothie with Wheatgerm	VEGETARIAN	74
Blueberry Smoothie	GLUTEN-FREE VEGAN	75
Almond Milk Smoothie	GLUTEN-FREE VEGETARIAN	76
Turmeric Ginger Smoothie	GLUTEN-FREE VEGETARIAN	77
Peanut Butter and Banana Shake	GLUTEN-FREE VEGETARIAN	78

Salads — 81

Asparagus and Green Bean Salad	GLUTEN-FREE	82
Iceberg Wedge Salad with Blue Cheese Dressing	GLUTEN-FREE	83
Chinese Chicken Salad		84
Udon Noodle Salad with Salmon		86
Seared Salmon and Chickpea Salad	GLUTEN-FREE	88
Spring Vegetable Quinoa Salad	VEGAN	89
Light Avocado Chicken Salad		90
Mango Chicken Salad	GLUTEN-FREE	91
Apricot Caprese Salad	GLUTEN-FREE VEGETARIAN	92
Waldorf Salad	GLUTEN-FREE VEGETARIAN	93
Tuna Potato Salad	GLUTEN-FREE	94

Main Meals — 96

Cashew Chicken	GLUTEN-FREE	98
Chicken with Sauteed Mushrooms		100
Mango Tilapia	GLUTEN-FREE	101
Lentil burgers	VEGETARIAN	102
Black Bean Burgers	VEGETARIAN	103
Chicken and Red Potatoes		104
Steak and Blackberry Glaze	GLUTEN-FREE	106
Kung Pao Chicken	GLUTEN-FREE	108
Crispy Peanut Shrimp		110
Pork Chops and Apples	GLUTEN-FREE	111
Carbonara		112
Papaya Whitefish with Ginger		113
Tomato Sauce-Free Lasagna		114
Turkey Meatballs		116
Quinoa Stuffed Chicken Roll-Ups	GLUTEN-FREE	117
Glazed Salmon and Lentils	GLUTEN-FREE	118
Pecan Crusted Trout	GLUTEN-FREE	119
Mac and Cheese with Salmon		120
Chicken Parmesan		121
Juicy Turkey and Mushroom Burgers		122
Buttermilk Chicken		123

Chicken Tetrazzini		124
Cauliflower Steak	GLUTEN-FREE VEGETARIAN	126
Shrimp and Pea Stir Fry		127
Creamy Mac and Cheese	VEGETARIAN	128
Fettuccine Alfredo	VEGETARIAN	129
Gnocchi	VEGETARIAN	130

Soups and Stew — 133

Chicken Noodle Soup		134
Eggplant Soup	GLUTEN-FREE VEGETARIAN	135
Chicken and Barley Stew	GLUTEN-FREE	136
Chicken and Black-Eyes Pea Soup	GLUTEN-FREE	137
Chickpea and Lentil Soup	GLUTEN-FREE VEGAN	138
Turkey White Bean Soup	GLUTEN-FREE	139
Butternut Soup	GLUTEN-FREE VEGAN	140

Snacks, Sides, and Extras — 143

Low Acid GERD-Friendly Tomato Sauce*	GLUTEN-FREE VEGAN	144
Basil Pesto	VEGETARIAN	145
Dill Oil	VEGAN	146
Ginger Mashed Potatoes	VEGETARIAN	147
Baked French Fries	VEGAN	148
Bok Choy Slaw	VEGAN	149
Parsnip French Fries	VEGAN	150
Stuffed Mushroom Caps		151
Sautéed Spinach with Apples and Walnuts	VEGAN	152
Crispy Quinoa	VEGAN	153
Artichoke and Spinach Dip	VEGETARIAN	154
Olive, Walnut, and Edamame Mix	VEGAN	155
Candied Pecans	VEGAN	156
Dried Persimmon	VEGAN	157
Ginger Tea	GLUTEN-FREE VEGAN	158

Desserts — 161

Healthy Apple Crisp	VEGETARIAN	162
Vanilla Almond Parfait	VEGETARIAN	163
Coconut rice pudding	VEGETARIAN	164

Chia Pudding With Honeydew Melon		VEGAN	165
Blueberry and Banana Sorbet		VEGAN	166
Watermelon Parfait		VEGETARIAN	167
Strawberry Sorbet	GLUTEN-FREE	VEGAN	168
Angel Food Cupcakes		VEGETARIAN	169
Crème Brûlée		VEGETARIAN	

Errore. Il segnalibro non è definito.

Arroz con Leche		VEGETARIAN	172
Flan	GLUTEN-FREE	VEGETARIAN	174
Sweet Potato Tarts		VEGETARIAN	176
Papaya, Yogurt. and Walnut Boat		VEGETARIAN	178

Conclusion 180

Others books by Robert Dickens 181

Dear Reader

One day I asked myself, how is it that after people have tried every type of prescription medication and treatment, still they cannot get rid of their symptoms?

My name is Robert, I am a researcher and I have always tried to help people understand how to treat their diseases in an all-natural way. By all-natural I mean changing diet and starting to gain awareness about one's own body.

Your journey towards a cure, does not involve the usage of any prescription medication nor the purchase of costly products. My goal is to make people understand how their bodies work in a simple way, and to make them understand the causes of their symptoms. Traditional medicine does not take into consideration the cause, or the origin of diseases, but rather it focuses on the symptoms, alleviating them with prescription medications.

With this book, I do not intend to tell anyone to stop using their prescription medication, but rather offer a second point of view on how to approach a cure starting from nutrition.

This is the reason I suggest you follow this book, if you are looking to cure you acid reflux. The information you find in this book comes directly from my research and other doctors' research, which is focused on helping people take care of their health, and understand the causes of mild conditions such as acid reflux.

I would like to thank my wife, Anita who helped me write this book. Together we were able to include easy and affordable recipes, that you will be able to follow in a 28-day meal plan. My wife is not a chef, however, she loves to cook, therefore, these recipes will truly be easy to make by anyone.

A warm thanks from

Robert & Anita

Introduction

Anyone who thinks that acid reflux is not a big deal has clearly never suffered from it! That is great for them. But for those who have suffered with it, we know how inconvenient and uncomfortable it can be. Sometimes it can be downright unbearable. My guess is that you have experienced acid reflux at least a few times in your lifetime. Picking up this book means that you are looking for a solution and a way not to let your acid reflux get in the way of your everyday life.

We all want to be free to live our lives without the pain that comes from acid reflux. It's not only painful but inconvenient. Having to excuse yourself in the middle of a family gathering to deal with heartburn is not ideal. Sometimes it's not even just a quick thing as symptoms can last up to two hours. Nobody wants to be uncomfortable or in pain for that long.

The good news is that you don't have to continue suffering indefinitely. While acid reflux may not have a cure, there are definitely things you can do to ease and manage the symptoms so that you can live a much more comfortable life. I have also suffered from heartburn. So, I am speaking from a place of experience when I say that there are ways to improve the quality of your life. I have tried many different things to ease heartburn, and I can confidently say that I am far better off now than before.

I am incredibly happy that you picked up this book. It means that you are ready to do something about your acid reflux. There are so many people out there that suffer in silence or who ignore the symptoms of acid reflux. The worst thing you could do is just ignore it. It could lead to worse problems down the line. It is not something to be ashamed of. There are hundreds of thousands of people who suffer from this around the globe.

Getting the right information is the first step on your journey to a happier, healthier, and more comfortable life. This book is not only filled with information about acid reflux but also with recipes and a 28-day meal plan. The hardest thing about lifestyle change is getting started. I wanted to make the process a bit easier by giving you the information you need to kick-start your journey. You can just jump in without the need for an intense planning session.

This book is not meant to be a fact sheet or just a recipe book, but a lifestyle guide. You should come out fully equipped with the information you need to create a new lifestyle that is more beneficial to you. Because of this, we can't just jump into the how to's. You have to understand what acid reflux is, what causes it, and what you can do to manage it. It's like building up a foundation. You have to start with the basics and build up your core knowledge before jumping into meal planning, shopping, and cooking the meals. Now, let's begin this journey by jumping straight into the basics.

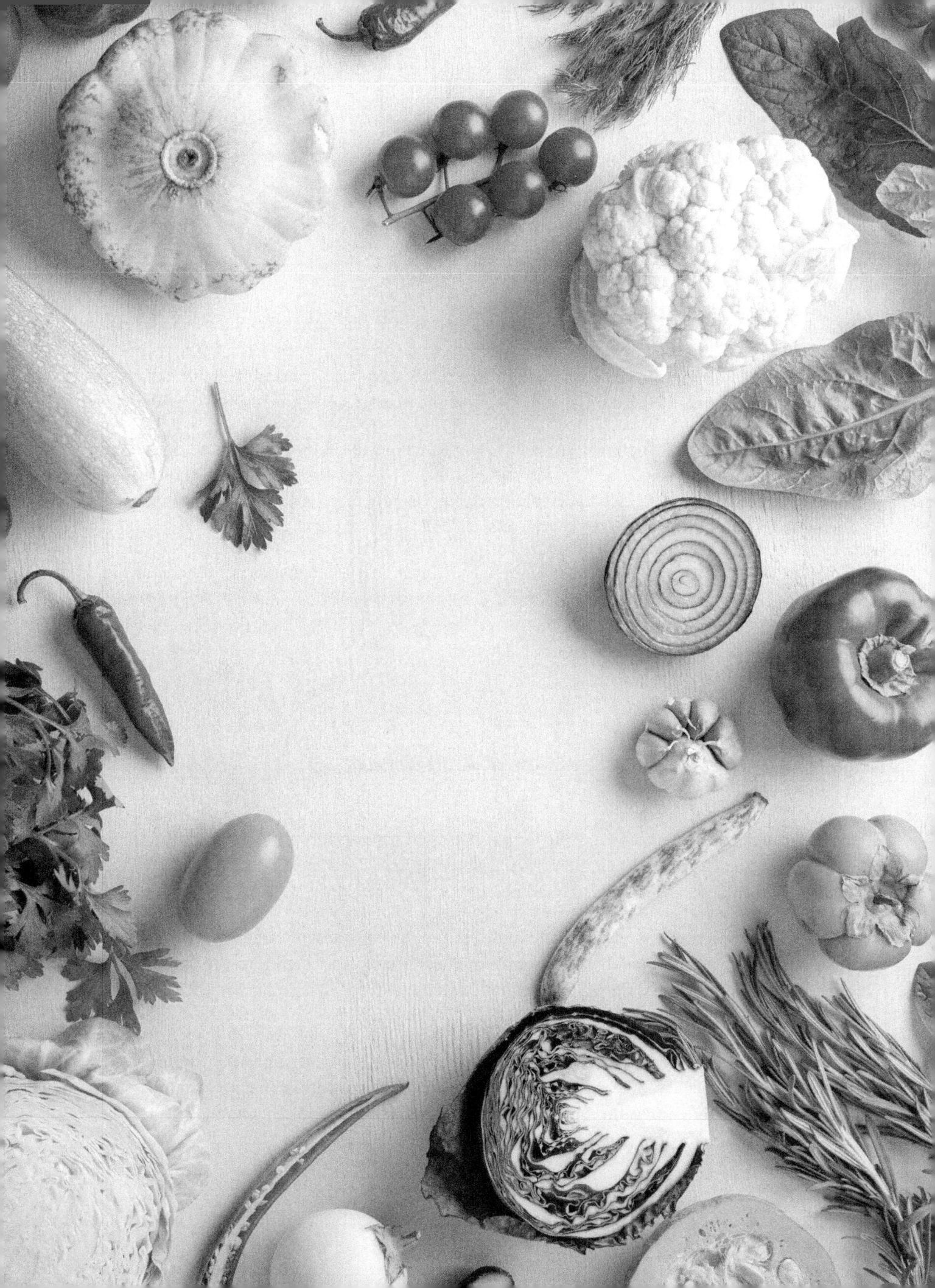

Chapter 1

The Basics of Acid Reflux

If you have ever suffered a burning pain in your lower chest, then you have acid reflux. Acid reflux is a prevalent problem in the western world. If you do suffer from it, then there is no need to feel alone. In fact, over 60 million people in America suffer from heartburn about once a month (MacGill, 2017). That is a substantial amount of people that are going through this regularly.

Acid reflux happens when acid from the stomach comes back up the esophagus. This is what causes that burning sensation. It is also often referred to as heartburn even though it is not happening in the heart itself. The acid that comes up the food pipe is used in the stomach to break down food. The stomach is built to handle this acid, but the esophagus is not.

Whether you have experienced this only a few times or it is a constant thing in your life, it is not a nice feeling. The good news is that there are things you can do about it. The best thing you can do to prepare is to get the most amount of knowledge. Once you can recognize the signs, you will be able to implement the remedies.

Signs of Acid Reflux

Acid reflux can be a once in a while thing, or it could happen very often. If you suffer from acid reflux more than twice a week, you have gastroesophageal reflux disease (GERD). In western countries, GERD affects between 20 to 30 percent of the population (MacGill, 2017).

The primary symptoms of acid reflux are pain or burning in your chest, discomfort in your throat, and the regurgitation of acid in your mouth or throat. Other signs are a feeling of a lump in your throat or difficulty swallowing. You would often feel these symptoms are eating a meal, and they worsen when you lie down.

There are also a few symptoms that are not as common, but you might also experience them. These are chronic cough, new asthma, and disrupted sleep patterns. These symptoms show up when you suffer from acid reflux at night. Night-time acid reflux is quite common because you will be lying down, causing it to flare up.

Should I Ignore Acid Reflux?

If you suffer from acid reflux, then you know it is not a pleasant experience. The thing is that many people will just leave it to pass and carry on with their lives. Sure, you could do this if you only have acid reflux once in a while. But if it is a frequent occurrence, it should definitely not be ignored.

Most people will experience acid reflux and heartburn at some point in their lives. In these cases, you can just let it pass or take an over the counter medication if you really want to. When it happens more often, then you should take action. The only parts of our bodies that are designed to handle acid are in the lower digestive system. Our esophaguses are just not made to hold acid, and that is why it burns. This could also lead to damage to our esophagus.

If you leave acid reflux untreated, it could lead to bleeding, swallowing problems, inflammation, and even cancer. The acid that comes up might even start eroding your teeth. Ulcers could form in the throat, or you might develop an esophageal stricture. A stricture happens when there is scarring in the esophagus caused by the acid. When the scar tissue builds up, it causes the esophagus to get narrower, causing problems swallowing food and drink. This is usually fixed through a procedure where the esophagus is stretched out.

Another common problem that we see with people who suffer from chronic acid reflux is Barrett's esophagus. About 5 to 10 percent of people who suffer from GERD have Barrett's esophagus. This disease causes precancerous changes to happen to the cells in the esophagus. There are very few symptoms, and they are not apparent. So, it is best to get yourself checked out if you do suffer from GERD. The doctor will be able to remove the abnormal cells if they diagnose it early.

If you have pain in your throat, you should consult with your doctor. It is always better to be safe than sorry. Once these things start to develop, you will need medical help to heal what was damaged. Your doctor will be able to point you in the right direction, give you medication, or even book you in for a procedure. They will have a better idea of what is going on. Therefore, if you are ever in doubt, seek out medical advice.

This section is not meant to scare you. The goal is to be honest and let you know the possible consequences of ignoring your acid reflux. You never want to get to the point where you have to go in for a massive medical procedure. This potential outcome is why it is so important not to ignore acid reflux. The sooner you make lifestyle changes and seek help and advice, the better. Most of the time, people can avoid these drastic situations with a few changes in lifestyle and diet.

10 Important Things to Know if You Suffer From Acid Reflux

Is it true that 8 glasses of water per day are good for you?

The reason there is not a scientific study about this theory, is something to think about. Moreover, we observe that people have difficulties drinking 8 glasses of water per day, this is because our body refuse it.

So, how much water should we drink?

To simplify, we could say that it is recommended to drink 8 glasses of liquids per day, keeping into consideration what we eat as well. To give some examples: a watermelon slice contains 95% of water, the same goes for vegetable soup, but even pasta that at first might seem a dry food, actually gains water throughout the cooking process.

With these few pieces of information, you might have guessed that it is not actually required to drink water during meals. In fact, my suggestion is not to drink during meals, especially if you suffer from acid reflux. There is not a fixed rule about how much to drink, however I can give you some useful indications:

- First, if you suffer from acid reflux, reduce the amount of liquids you drink throughout the day.

- If you eat a meal full of fruits and vegetables, drink a small amount of water.

- If you eat foods containing lots of water such as: watermelon, broth, vegetable soup etc., avoid drinking water or any other drink.

- If you eat dry foods such as: pizza, crackers, croissant etc., drink 2 cups of water at most. These foods will absorb the water and will swell in the stomach, like a sponge. This reaction will favor acid reflux because in the stomach there won't be enough space for both, food and gastric juices.

- Drink outside meals as much as possible, I will explain the reason further ahead.

Now I would like to touch on the reason why drink lots of liquids could favor acid reflux.

It is a simple mechanic action: if while eating we introduce first solid food and then water, this last one will be blocked and it will create a clog in the stomach, which may disrupt the digestive process.

Afterwards, the gastric juices will pour into the stomach as well and will be diluted in the water, since they will stay longer in the stomach, the gastric juices will create some toxic gases, that will cause discomfort, since these gases will start to rise and inflame the cardiac sphincter, and, in worse cases they will cause a hiatal hernia.

I just described a very discomforting situation, that I believe you might be already familiar with, since you are reading this book. It is for this exact reason that earlier I suggested to drink outside of meals, so that the liquids can pass quickly through the stomach and will not be blocked by the solid food.

I truly wanted to give you this piece of advice, since it is so simple, yet many doctors do not take it into consideration.

This is an example of acid reflux caused by drinking too much liquids

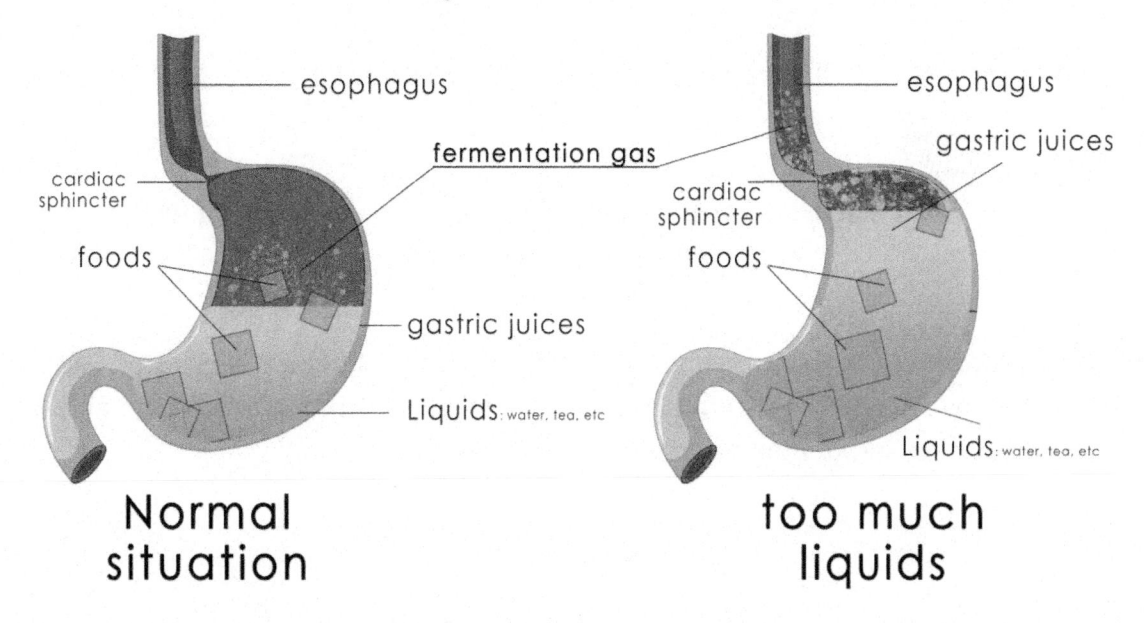

Normal situation
- esophagus
- cardiac sphincter
- foods
- fermentation gas
- gastric juices
- Liquids: water, tea, etc

too much liquids
- esophagus
- gastric juices
- cardiac sphincter
- foods
- Liquids: water, tea, etc

Can sleep alleviate acid reflux?

More than sleep in itself, the position in which a person lays down might be significant. To people that ask me this question I tell them to avoid laying down facing upwards, since it will not be beneficial for digestion. It is preferable to lay on the side, the best option will be laying on the right side.

In fact, laying on the right side will help the correct functioning of the digestive system. In this position, each organ is relaxed and not compromised by gravity. This is also the reason why when a doctor is performing an enema asks patients to lay on one side. Moreover, we can refer to nature as well, other mammals rarely sleep on their back, they rather sleep on their side, we can observe this phenomenon taking monkeys as an example.

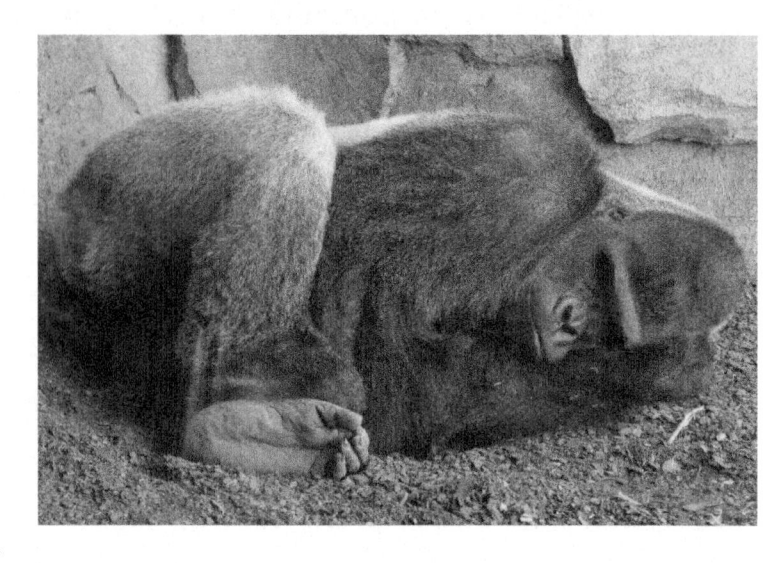

It is important to eat food at the right temperature

Often, in our busy lives, we might have not enough time to correctly warm up our lunches. Unfortunately, eating cold food could favor acid reflux, in fact cold temperatures irritate the stomach making it lazier, whether warmer temperatures will help stretch out the stomach and making it more productive.

This does not mean that every food needs to be eaten warm, you can follow this rule:

Each food that has been cooked, always has to be eaten warm.

Therefore, cooked vegetables, pasta, rice, meat, pizza etc., always need to be eaten warm to digest correctly and to avoid acid reflux. On the other hand, fruits and raw vegetables, including jams can be consumed at room temperature.

Can recipes in this book help me treat my acid reflux?

Of course! These recipes realized with my wife Anita, are studied to alleviate the discomfort caused by acid reflux. However, I would like to clarify one thing, each person is unique, therefore recipes in this book might not work for everyone. I always tell my patients to listen to the guidelines given by doctors but also to think with their own head. If a diet is not working for you, always ask yourself questions, if a prescription medication is making you uncomfortable, always ask why is that. Unlikely to what we have been told, I believe each therapy should vary from person to person.

To give an obvious example, these recipes are useful to reduce acid reflux, however, if while following the meal plan, you keep drinking lots of water, following this diet will be less effective.

Recently I have been following some studies conducted by an Italian doctor, Dr. Pietro Mozzi, who discovered a relationship between nutrition and blood types. This example is connected to what I was explaining earlier, that every person reacts differently depending on what one eats.

Dr. Mozzi explains that if a person whose blood type is A would eat red meat, that person's acid reflux will be worse than a person eating the same meat but whose blood type is O, who instead could be potentially cured from acid reflux. Another example could be pumpkin, which can enhance acid reflux in people with blood type B but, won't have any effect on people with other blood types. Another thing to take into consideration are some combos that could be harmful for people with certain blood types; for example if a person with blood type A eats a potato and tomato soup, will experience a very bad stomach ache. Another thing to avoid would be the pumpkin-starch mix (e.g. rice, wheat pasts, etc.) this too could cause acid reflux.

Right now I will not talk into blood types in details, it might be an interesting topic for a future book. My suggestion is the following:

You should start knowing your own body, understanding what foods are good and what are bad for you. Each person is unique.

Complications Caused By Acid Reflux

Continuous acid reflux might actually be GERD. GERD is a chronic disease that needs management. If left untreated, then it could lead to ulcers, bleeding, or esophageal cancer. It is important to note that you are not at risk of anything serious if you have a small amount of acid reflux over a period of time. You are only at risk of these when you are continually having acid reflux, which is then diagnosed as GERD.

One particular thing about red meat in this diet that no one else will tell you

As previously mentioned, the studies conducted by Dr. Mozzi are having interesting developments in the relationship between blood type and nutrition. One proven relationship is the affinity between red meats and people whose blood type is O. It has always been known that in order to reduce acid reflux, red meats should have been avoided. This statement is true, however, not for people with blood type O. In fact, these people are naturally predispose to eating meat, if these people would eat red meat, their discomfort given by acid reflux might be alleviated and in some cases it will even disappear.

Therefore, if your blood type is O, and you love red meat, you will be able to eat it with no consequences, as long as you will not fry or cook the meat in butter or oil, but simply cook it on the grill.

Try to believe!

Anita's advice is to cook red meat with red wine of your choice. I tried it and it was delicious!

You can eat legumes, but pay attention to one thing...

Legumes do not cause acid reflux, nonetheless, you would need to pay attention to one thing if you wish to keep your digestive system healthy. Legumes should not be mixed with starchy foods. This is because the mixture of these two will cause a bloating and gassy feeling. If the gases reach the stomach it might favor acid reflux. Therefore, legumes cannot be mixed with starchy foods or even among themselves.

Just one type of legume per meal.

If you suffer from IBS I recommend my books:

- ***Low FODMAP diet cookbook:*** *101 Easy, healthy & fast recipes for yours low-FODMAP diet*
- ***Low FODMAP diet****: The Beginner's Guide*

Acid Reflux Can Be Linked to Diet

I have mentioned that GERD is most common in western countries. The reason for this is the diet we eat. Because this is a gut issue, it definitely can be linked to the foods we eat. This is not always the case, so it is important to note that you can have a perfectly healthy diet but still have some acid reflux. Many different things can cause this from pregnancy to smoking.

Usually, acidic and fatty foods can be triggers for acid reflux. When acidic foods hit your stomach, they could immediately trigger acid reflux. This is because acid reflux is the bringing up of acid. Fatty foods have a different effect, but it still leads to bringing acid back up. Fatty foods lower the ant reflux barrier in your gut. This occurrence increases the chance of you having acid reflux.

Treatment Can Vary

Every person is different and will respond to different treatments. Above this, some people prefer to do things a certain way, while others prefer alternative methods. All this should be taken into account when picking the treatment you want to go for. For someone who only experiences acid reflux on an occasional basis, you could identify trigger foods and avoid them. Some people prefer the over the counter approach by getting antacids and taking them when they feel the reflux coming on or before they eat something that could trigger acid reflux. Your doctor could also prescribe chronic medication or some other solution based on your situation. In extreme cases, a doctor might suggest surgery on the valve that creates the reflux.

Losing Lots of Weight Is Not Necessary

While acid reflux can be linked to obesity, it is unnecessary to lose an extreme amount of weight to stop it. This does not mean that you shouldn't lose any weight at all. Losing 10 to 15 pounds may be all that is needed to help with acid reflux. The goal should be to return to your baseline weight. Baseline weight is the weight you were before you started suffering from heartburn. So don't feel like you need to become a certain weight or drop everything all at once. Focus on getting back to where you were before the acid reflux started, and then you can continue working from there. At this point, you will already start feeling better.

At Home, Natural Remedies

If you require an effective at-home remedy for heartburn, you should give these a try. These remedies may not offer long-term relief, but they can help ease the discomfort. Not all of them may work for you, so give them a try and see which one is the best fit.

Baking Soda

Baking soda is a natural acid neutralizer. Please make sure that you are using baking soda and not baking powder. Baking powder is affordable, and you can find it in almost every grocery store. All you need to do is dissolve it in a glass of water and drink it. You may have to skip this remedy if you are on a low sodium diet. Baking soda does contain sodium so just be aware of that.

Ginger Tea

Ginger root has a lot of medicinal properties and can help soothe the stomach. You can either buy a caffeine-free ginger tea or make one on your own. I would suggest making it yourself because you can be sure it is pure ginger and nothing else. There is a simple recipe for ginger tea in the recipe section under the heading "drinks."

Aloe Juice

Only for people with blood type A

Aloe juice can be found at most grocery stores and is quite affordable. Try and find one that is all-natural and does not contain any preservatives. The fewer ingredients, the better. You can have about ½ a cup before meals to help soothe your esophagus. Aloe water and aloe juice are not the same things, so make sure you are getting the right product. Aloe water is usually very diluted and will not have the same effect as pure aloe juice.

Banana

Eating a banana is one of the oldest and most relied-upon methods to ease heartburn. Bananas contain natural antacids. If you start your day by eating a banana, it really helps counteract the effects of acid reflux.

FAQ

Does Everyone Who Has Acid Reflux Have GERD?

Not necessarily. Many people have acid reflux and do have GERD, but this is not the majority. The chances of you experiencing acid reflux a few times in your life are pretty high. If you only suffer from heartburn once or twice a month, then this is not GERD. It may be caused by the food you ate. The best thing you can do is monitor the foods you are eating just before you get heartburn. Monitoring your foods will help you pinpoint what you should be avoiding.

Can Children Develop GERD?

Yes, people of all ages can have acid reflux and GERD. This includes babies. In fact, more than half of all babies under the age of three months have GERD (Cunha, 2017). Many babies have tummy issues that cause gas, diarrhea, and constipation. GERD is just the moving of the stomach contents back up the esophagus, and we often do see this in children and babies. The most common symptoms of GERD in children are frequent vomiting, persistent coughing, not wanting to eat, heartburn, and pain in the abdomen (stomach area).

Is There a Cure for GERD?

There is no permanent cure for GERD. Once you have it, it will be something you will have to manage for the rest of your life. The good news is that you can manage it and drastically reduce the symptoms and the amount you suffer. This is done through the remedies mentioned above as well as changing your diet, some over the counter medication, and surgery (if you want to go that route).

Who Has a High Risk of Developing GERD?

There are many reasons someone may contract GERD. There are some instances where you suffer from it and cannot find a particular cause. With that being said, if you are pregnant, obese, or a smoker you, are at higher risk of developing GERD or acid reflux in general.

Chapter 2

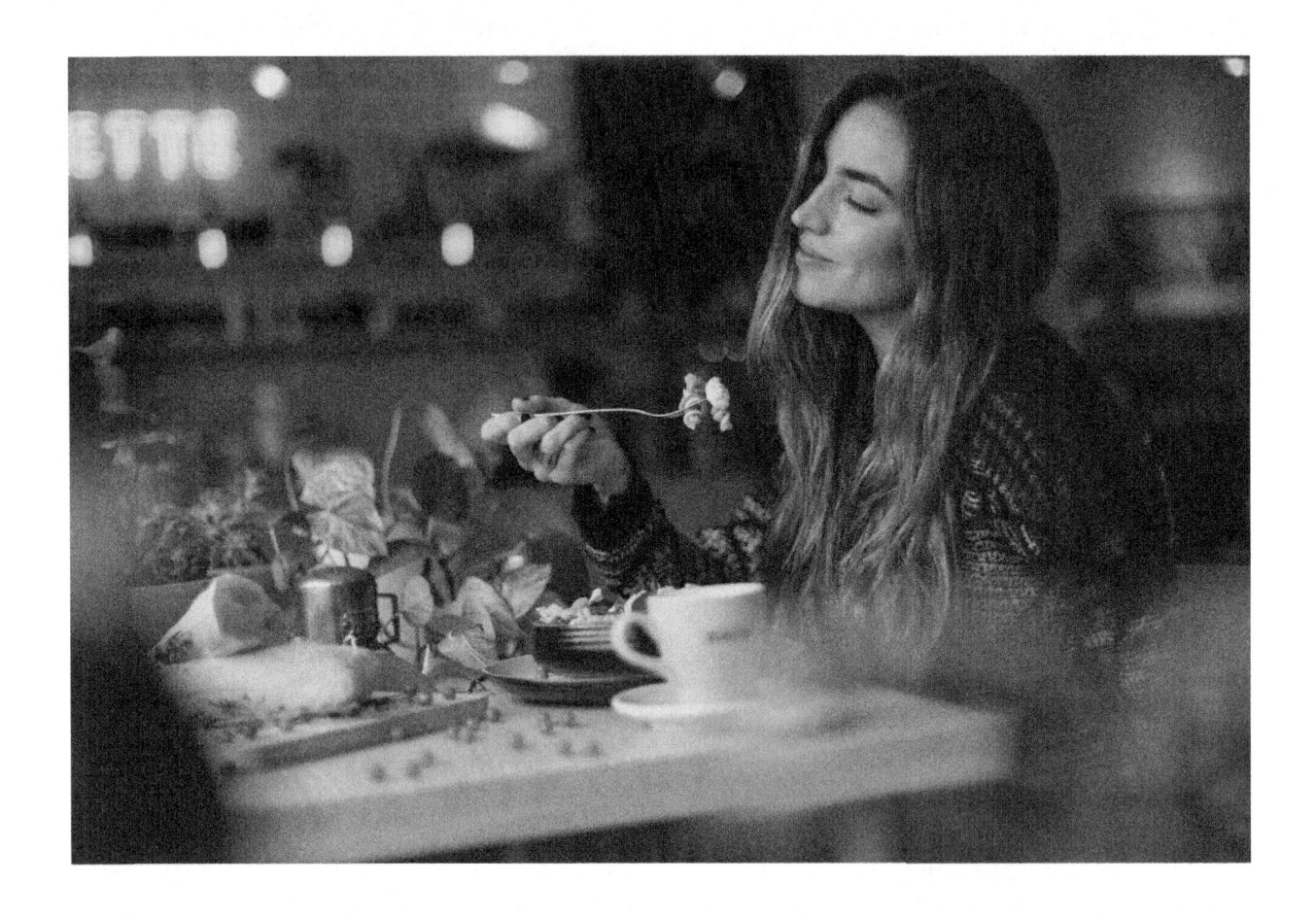

Eating for Acid Reflux

Acid reflux is definitely not an enjoyable experience. It is uncomfortable and is just not ideal. Luckily, some foods can help you avoid and relieve the symptoms of acid reflux. In the same way, there are foods that can trigger acid reflux and make it worse.

The best thing you can do is understand what foods trigger your acid reflux and what foods relieve the symptoms. Everybody is different, so there may be some foods that cause acid reflux that are not on this list. You need to do some of your own testing, and you will learn through trial and error.

Start by adding the foods that are good for you and slowly removing the trigger foods. Keeping a food diary is very helpful for this. You can write down what you are eating each day and track what foods you have eaten that may be linked to acid reflux. Doing so will help you get a better idea of what foods you should be avoiding. Take a look at the list below to get a better idea of the foods that are good for you and the ones that you should avoid.

What to Eat

The below foods will help you manage the symptoms of acid reflux. When you feel the acid reflux coming on, try and eat one or some of these foods to help you. Some may work better for you than others, so don't get discouraged if you eat something and don't feel a huge difference. Eventually, you will find the foods that work the best for you.

Vegetables

We all know that vegetables are good for us. If anything, adding more vegetables to your diet will increase the amount of nutrients your body is getting. They are naturally low in fat and acid. Some good options are leafy green vegetables, potatoes, cucumber, broccoli, and cauliflower.

Ginger

Please don't think that you have to chomp down on a whole thumb of ginger. Thankfully you do not need a lot of it to gain the benefits. A great way to incorporate ginger into your diet is to add sliced or crushed pieces to your food or smoothies. You could also make ginger tea. Ginger is a natural anti-inflammatory food and is very good for many gastrointestinal problems.

Oats

Anything high in fiber is beneficial for your digestive system and can help relieve acid reflux. Oats are easy to make and have a lot of fiber in it. You can easily incorporate it into your diet by having it for breakfast with fruit.

Non-citrus fruit

Fruit is generally very good for you, so you will do your body good if you increase the amount you eat. Citrus is high in acid, and that is why you should be avoiding those types of fruit. Some of the fruit that you can incorporate into your diet are **bananas, apples, melons, and pears.**

Lean meat and seafood

The key word here is lean. These types of meats are low in fat and high in protein. Some examples of these foods are seafood, turkey, and chicken. Cooking them by grilling, poaching, and baking is best. Always avoid frying.

Egg Whites

The entire egg is filled with nutrients and protein, but the yolk is also high in fat. This could trigger acid reflux. Sticking to just the whites is a great way to get in the protein without the added fat.

Healthy Fats

Good fats can actually help with acid reflux. It is the saturated and trans fats that cause a significant problem. While it is not good to eat large amounts of any fat, healthy fats are packed full of nutrients and can help lessen the symptoms of acid reflux. Sources of healthy fats include avocados, nuts, flaxseed, and olive oil.

What to Avoid

There has been some debate around what food causes acid reflux. However, certain foods have been shown to cause acid problems in many people. You may have noticed that when you eat a certain food, you get heartburn. While the food might not be the only cause for acid reflux, it definitely can be a trigger. Avoiding anything that could make your body unhappy is key to controlling the symptoms. Take a look at this list of common trigger foods and see if there is anything you have experienced problems with.

Fatty foods

This is a broad category, but I'm sure there were a few foods that popped into your mind when you read that. Fried foods, fast food, full-fat dairy, and fatty meats are all included. Fatty foods delay the stomach from emptying and cause stomach acid to back up. It is better to avoid these foods as much as you can. They generally cause more harm than good.

Citrus fruit and tomatoes

These are very acidic fruits and are not suitable for people who suffer from acid-related problems. Do your best to avoid them. Some of the fruit on the list are oranges, lemons, and pineapples. If you are worried that you won't be able to have a delicious tomatoey sauce ever again, then take a look at our low-acid tomato sauce in the recipe section.

Spicy food

These foods won't cause reflux in every person, but it can cause problems for some. It is best to track what happens to your body when you eat foods like this. Sometimes it is the specific way it's cooked or the dish itself that's the problem, not the whole category of food.

Caffeine and mint

It has been reported that some people suffer from acid reflux after they have a cup of coffee or chewed on a piece of mint gum. If you notice this, then try and avoid these two things. Instead, go for caffeine-free coffee and mint-free gum and sweets.

Chocolate

This is a food that most people would be sad to avoid. Unfortunately, chocolate has been shown to increase acid reflux due to the presence of something called methylxanthine.

What to Drink

We already know that drinks high in caffeine, highly acidic drinks, and carbonated drinks are not good for acid reflux. However, we haven't spoken about the types of drinks that you should consume. Do not overlook this. Now you should not be drinking too many liquids as this could cause your acid reflux to flare up, but many drinks are very good for you.

Herbal teas

Herbal teas are great for aiding digestion and are used for various digestive problems. Chamomile, licorice, and ginger teas are the best for acid reflux. They calm the stomach and can help soothe you. Just remember to avoid mint teas.

Smoothies

These are definitely a great way to get added nutrients into your diet. The best part is that you can add ingredients that will help soothe your heartburn. Bananas, apples, ginger, and non-citrus fruits are all great options. Smoothies are easy to digest, easy to swallow, and are very cooling when they go down. Having a smoothie with the right ingredients can help with acid reflux and its symptoms.

Fruit juices

We have already spoken about avoiding citrus fruits in your diet, but citrus fruits are not the only fruit that makes great juices. There are plenty of non-citrus fruits that can be juiced. One of the best ways to get your fruit juice is cold-pressed juices. These retain their nutrients and are free from unnecessary ingredients and flavorings. You can buy them in the shops or buy a juicer and juice your own fruit and veggies. Some great options are carrot and ginger, aloe vera, watermelon, and cucumber.

Water

We should all be getting enough water into our diets. The PH of water is neutral, which means it can help raise the PH of an acidic meal. Drinking too much water can have adverse effects on acid reflux, so don't overdo it. If you drink when you are thirsty, you should be fine. It is best not to overthink this one.

Food Swaps

Food swaps are one of the best ways to transition into a new diet or way of eating. We all have our favorites, and sometimes it can be hard to give certain things up. Food swapping allows you to use something similar in the place of the food or ingredients you love. Let's take a look at some food swaps you can make in your everyday life.

Coffee for Herbal Tea

There are many coffee drinkers out there, but unfortunately, the caffeine makes it bad for those who suffer from acid reflux. If you still want a nice warm drink, try going for herbal teas rather. They are much easier on the stomach, and many of them actually aid in digestion. You can add some milk to it for a creamier drink if you are not happy with just the tea and water.

Once you get used to drinking tea, you won't even miss the coffee. It is just a matter of pushing through until you no longer crave coffee. Remember that caffeine is addictive, and that is why so many people struggle to give up coffee. If you are someone who has coffee multiple times a day, then you might have to either wean yourself off it or suffer from a few withdrawal symptoms before you can go without it. Don't be disheartened if it is a bit hard at the beginning. You will eventually not even miss it.

Citrus Fruit for Berries and Melons

The reason so many people love citrus fruit is that they are so juicy and sweet. Fortunately, there are plenty of other fruits that have the same characteristics. They may not taste the same, but melons and berries are juicy and delicious. Fill your fridge and fruit basket with these fruits instead of citrus fruits.

I would go as far as to say that berries and melons are much better than citrus fruits in terms of variety and usability. You can cook with berries much easier and transform them in your dishes. Using them as garnishes and toppings is also a great idea. Smoothies with these fruits are also super delicious. The possibilities are endless.

Chocolate for Carob Powder or Alkalized Cocoa

I think giving up chocolate is one that makes many people who suffer from acid reflux very sad. Almost everyone enjoys a block of chocolate. The thing is, chocolate is both high in fat and acidic. That is a double trigger, which is why it is best just to give it a skip if you suffer from acid reflux. If you can have a block now and then without it triggering heartburn, then by all means, go for it. Just be careful and don't overdo it.

If you really need a chocolate fix, then try

carob powder or alkalized cocoa. Alkalized cocoa is also called Dutch-processed powder and is more alkaline than acidic. This makes it safe for people who suffer from acid reflux. Carob powder is not related to cocoa at all and comes from the carob pod. It has very similar flavors to cocoa and you can use it in any recipe that asks for cocoa.

Now it is not a smart idea to just grab a spoonful of these powders and eat it straight. They will have a very bitter taste. You need to add them to the dishes. Chocolate cakes and desserts can be made using either of these two, and that should satisfy your chocolate craving.

Fried Food for Baked Food

Fried food is generally bad for everyone, even if they don't suffer from acid reflux. The high fat content is a massive contributor to weight gain, and it is also a trigger for acid reflux. It is best to give fried foods a skip and try and cut it out of your diet as much as you can.

You can bake basically anything that you can fry. Since it is the method of cooking that is changing here, you don't have to change the actual foods you are eating. There are plenty of recipes out there that turn the regular friend foods into healthy, baked alternatives. Some of these recipes are in the recipe section of this book so give them a try.

High Fat Dairy for Plant-Based Options

Dairy products are also a common acid reflux trigger. Again this can be a hard one for people to give up since it seems almost to be a staple in everybody's home. The good news is that there are plenty of plant-based dairy alternatives. These are easy to get at supermarkets, and many of them are not too expensive either.

Milk alternatives are soy milk, almond milk, and oat milk. Instead of regular yogurt, go for coconut yogurt. You can use all of these as direct substitutes for typical dairy products. So that makes it easy to add to your favorite recipes. If you are looking for a cheese substitute, you can get vegan cheese. It is more expensive than regular cheese. But if you want a sprinkle of cheese, it is an option. You can also add a bit of nutritional yeast for a cheesy flavor to your meal.

Tomato Pasta Sauce for Pesto

Tomato sauces on pasta are classic, but that is not the only way to enjoy pasta. Pesto is a great way to eat pasta, and it is delicious. You could also use some olive oil over your pasta for a more simple dish. Pasta is great with many things, so don't feel stuck because you are giving the red sauce a skip. You could also try making the low acid tomato sauce recipe in this book if you are craving some tomato paste. It is a great way to enjoy the red sauce still. Again, just be careful not to overdo it since not all the acid will be neutralized.

Garlic and Onions for Dried Versions

Although never eaten on their own, these two add a lot of flavor to food. Many dishes require one or both, so it can be difficult to get a flavorful dish without them. Instead of using fresh garlic and onions, try the dried variety. They are less likely to cause acid reflux. The other bonus is that you don't always have to be chopping onions or crushing garlic when you are making a meal.

There is a chance that the dried variety might still be a trigger for you. If this is the case, try using other herbs and spices for flavor. Basil, dill, and parsley add a lot of flavor to a variety of dishes. None of them taste like garlic or onion, but that does not mean that you won't be able to get a delicious tasting meal using them.

Alcohol for Non-Alcoholic Alternatives

Unfortunately, alcohol is a big acid reflux trigger, so it is best to avoid it altogether. If you are slightly tolerant, you can perhaps have one drink. However, be sure not to overdo it. It is important to know your limits as your health is the most important thing.

Thankfully, if you enjoy having a drink on certain occasions, there are alcohol-free options for you. You should still avoid Cconated beverages, so it will still not be a good idea to have non-alcoholic champagne and non-alcoholic beer. Rather, enjoy non-alcoholic wines and mocktails (which taste just like regular cocktails, but without the alcohol). In any case, you really don't need alcohol in your life. It isn't a staple, so don't feel like you are missing out because you can't have a drink.

Food List

Allowed	Allowed in limited quantities	Avoid
FRUITS		
APPLE (fresh, dried, juice)	PEACH	CITRUS FRUITS: (Lemon, Lime, Orange, Tangerine, Grapefruit)
BANANA	RASPBERRY	PINEAPPLE
MELON	GRAPES	CITRUS FRUITS JUICE
WATERMELON	APPLE CIDER	TOMATO
[Other fruits]	BLUEBERRY	POMEGRANATE
VEGETABLES		
ONION (powder)	GARLIC	TOMATO
GARLIC (powder)	LEEK	MINT
MUSHROOMS	SAUERKRAUT	FRIES
PEAS	SHALLOT	ONION (fresh)
SAUCE TOMATO	ONION (cooked, not fried)	CHIVE
LEGUMES	BELL PEPPER	CHILLI PEPPER
[other vegetables]		

CEREALS AND FLOURS

All cereals and bakery products are allowed except foods with **not** allowed ingredients such as: chocolate cookies, pasta with fat cheese, garlic bread, etc.

Allowed	Allowed in limited quantities	Avoid
DAIRY PRODUCTS		
[All kind of **low fat** dairy products even: sour cream]	YOGURT	ICE-CREAM
FETA	MILK	FRESH SOFT CHEESE
GOAT CHEESE	SKIMMED MILK	SOUR CREAM
TOFU	MOZZARELLA	MILK SHAKE
PHILADELPHIA	CHEDDAR CHEESE	MILK FLAKES
	GREEK YOGURT	

DRIED FRUIT AND SEEDS

All dried fruits and seeds are allowed:

WALNUTS, NUTS, PEANUTS, PEANUT BUTTER, CHIA, COCONUT GRATED DRIED, etc.

MEAT – FISH - EGGS

EGGS (not fried)	TUNE SALAD	ALL FRIED MEAT and FISH
LEAN MEAT: (chicken, turkey)	CHICKEN SALAD	RED MEAT
FRESH FISH	HAM	FATTY MEAT
CANNED FISH		

SWEETS AND FAT FOODS

LICORICE	KETCHUP	CHOCOLATE
NO FAT BISCUITS	LIGHT MAYONNAISE	CHIPS
HONEY	LOW FAT BISCUITS	CHOCOLATE COOKIES
STEVIA		INTINGOLI
MAPLE SYRUP		CHEWINGUM
RICE SYRUP		CANDIES

DRINKS

MILK: (almond, soy, coconut, oat)	LOW FAT MILK	COFFEE
FENNEL SEED TEA	BEER	WINE
CHAMOMILE	LEMONADE	TEA
WINE (for cooking)		LIQUOR
JUICE (allowed fruits)		CARBONATED DRINKS
HERBAL TEA		HOT CHOCOLATE

remember to drink a few liquids during the diet, even allowed drinks

CONDIMENTS

OIL (all)	APPLE VINEGAR	INTINGOLI
MISO	RICE VINEGAR	CITRUS JUICE
BARBECUE SAUCE	PAPRIKA	VINEGAR
MAPLE SYRUP		PEPPER (dark, white, etc)
TOMATO SAUCE		CHILLI PEPPER

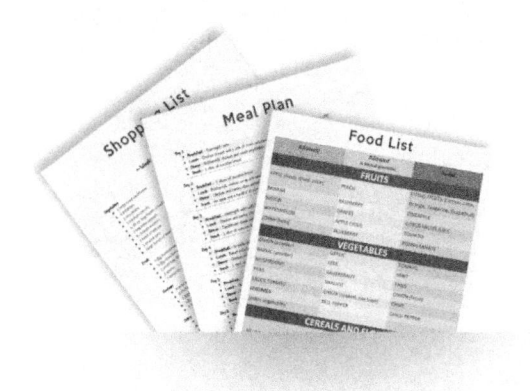

Chapter 3

Meal Plan and Shopping List

Planning and having the right things available to you will make eating the right way much more manageable. It is easier to eat something you are not supposed to if you feel like you have no other option. That is why planning in advance will help limit this from happening. You will always have something delicious to eat, but it will always be something that is good for you.

Building a Shopping List

The first step to making sure you have everything that you need is to have a shopping list. You need to know what you have and what you need to buy. This will stop you from buying unnecessary things and make sure you buy the things that you do need. It is also a great way to help you save some money. We often overestimate what we will need for the month when we don't have a list.

Meal planning before you go shopping for the week also helps you to buy the right things. If you know what you will be eating, you will know the ingredients you need for the meals. This measure is especially helpful when you are buying fresh produce. These things can go off very quickly, so buying too much is a waste.

With all this in mind, let's build a shopping list that will be beneficial to you. There are staples that you should always have in your cupboard, and then there are things you will need to buy every week. Here is an example of what you should be buying:

- Vegetables - leafy greens, broccoli, cauliflower, asparagus, carrots, potatoes, peas, beets, sweet potato, butternut squash, and sweet corn. Buying frozen veggies will allow you to buy in bulk and use them for longer.

- Fruit - Bananas, apples, pears, melon, apricots, plums, and coconut. Fruit is always best fresh, so you should buy this weekly.

- Whole grains - Bulgur, quinoa, brown rice, and rolled oats.

- Proteins - Chicken breast, fish, turkey mince, egg whites, lentils, and beans. You can go for red meat just make sure it is very lean and you don't eat it all the time.

- Herbs and spices - Brazil, oregano, rosemary, thyme and parsley. Most species shouldn't cause a problem, but avoid things like cayenne pepper and red pepper.

28 Day Meal Plan

This is a simple 28-day meal plan that you can follow. It will incorporate some classic, simple meals and some of the meals that you can be found in the recipe section. Breakfast, lunch, dinner, and snacks will all be covered, but you can also add a desert on the day you are feeling for a sweet treat.

The meals are easily interchangeable with other recipes that are found in the recipe section or any other recipe you might prefer. The main goal is to stick to the right types of foods. So, if you feel like swapping around meals, then go for it.

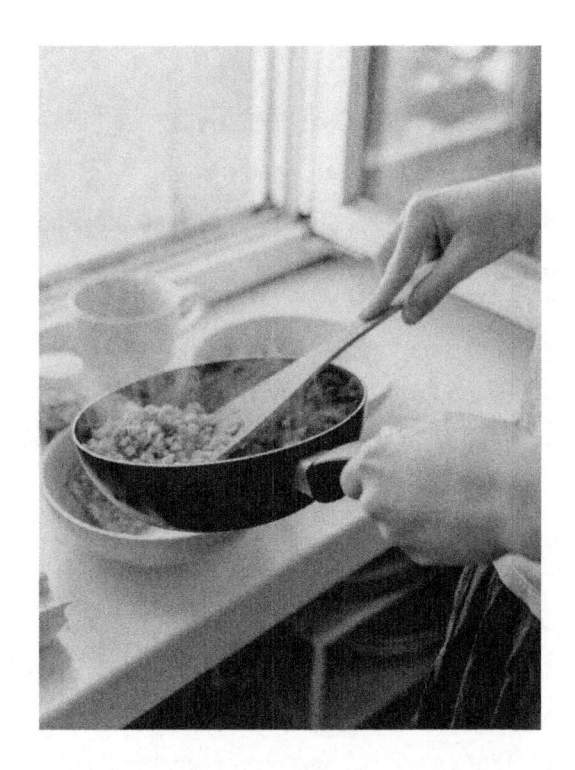

Day 1:
- **Breakfast** - Overnight oats — Pag. 52
- **Lunch** - Chicken breast and a side of roast potatoes — -
- **Dinner** - Buttermilk chicken and roast vegetables — Pag. 123
- **Snack** - 1 slice of zucchini bread — Pag. 60

Day 2:
- **Breakfast** - 2 slices of zucchini bread — Pag. 60
- **Lunch** - Buttermilk chicken wrap and salad — Pag. 123
- **Dinner** - Chicken and barley stew served over brown rice — Pag. 136
- **Snack** - An apple and a handful of strawberries — -

Day 3:
- **Breakfast** - Overnight oats with fruit — Pag. 52
- **Lunch** - Chicken and barley stew — Pag. 136
- **Dinner** - Cauliflower steak served with creamed spinach and mashed potatoes — Pag. 126
- **Snack** - 1 slice of zucchini bread — Pag. 60

Day 4:
- **Breakfast** - Granola and low-fat yogurt — Pag. 50
- **Lunch** - Baked potato with low-fat sour cream and shredded chicken — -
- **Dinner** - Chicken noodle soup — Pag. 134
- **Snack** - 1 slice of zucchini bread — Pag. 60

Day 5:
- **Breakfast** - Overnight oats — Pag. 52
- **Lunch** - Chicken noodle soup — Pag. 134
- **Dinner** - Roast chicken breast and roast vegetables — -
- **Snack** - 1 banana — -

Day 6:
- **Breakfast** - 2 slices of zucchini bread — Pag. 60
- **Lunch** - Chicken breast shredded on top of a garden salad — -
- **Dinner** - Turkey slices with roast vegetables and rice — -
- **Snack** - Apple slices and peanut butter — -

Day 7:
- **Breakfast** - Granola with low-fat yogurt — Pag. 50
- **Lunch** - Turkey slices and a side salad — -
- **Dinner** - Basil pesto and whole wheat pasta — Pag. 145
- **Snack** - 1 slice of zucchini bread — Pag. 60

~ Week 1 Shopping List ~

Vegetables:
- 1 large head cauliflower
- 4 potatoes
- 3 ribs celery
- 3 medium carrots,
- 1, 16 oz. bag frozen mixed vegetables
- 1 bag baby spinach
- 4 - 5 large zucchini
- 1 head of lettuce
- 1 oz pine nuts
- Large bunch of basil

Fruit:
- ½ lbs blueberries
- ½ lbs strawberries
- 1 small bag raisins
- 2 apples
- 2 bananas

Protein:
- 3 large eggs
- 6 chicken breasts
- 1 lbs bone-in, skin-on chicken thighs
- 1 lb boneless skinless chicken thighs
- 2 turkey breasts

Dairy:
- 1 block low-fat butter
- 1 litre milk of choice
- 32 oz nonfat Greek yogurt
- 1 can nonfat buttermilk
- 1 tub low-fat sour cream
- small bag grated parmesan cheese

Grains:
- ½ lbs barley
- 1 small bag brown rice
- ¼ cup dried pumpkin seeds
- 1 large bag rolled oats
- 3 lbs wheat germ
- 6 oz egg noodles

Condiments:
- ⅛ teaspoon hot sauce
- 1 jar peanut butter

Sweeteners:
- ½ lbs sugar
- 2 teaspoons light brown sugar
- 3 teaspoon honey
- 3 teaspoon vanilla

Herbs and Spices:
- 1 bottle garlic powder
- 1 bottle onion powder
- 2 teaspoons Italian seasoning
- 2 bay leaves
- 1 tablespoon ground cinnamon
- ¼ teaspoon ground nutmeg
- ¼ teaspoon ground cloves
- ½ teaspoon dried tarragon
- 1 teaspoon dried rosemary
- 1 tablespoon Dried oregano
- 1 tablespoon Dried thyme
- 1 bag salt
- 1 bunch fresh parsley

Liquids:
- 2, 32 oz cartons low-sodium chicken broth
- 2 tablespoons white wine vinegar

Oils:
- 1 bottle canola oil
- 1 bottle olive oil

Dry Baking Ingredients:
- Baking powder
- Baking soda
- 1 large bag all-purpose white flour
- 1 small bag whole wheat flour

Day 8:
- **Breakfast** - Strawberry banana smoothie — Pag. 67
- **Lunch** - Chicken breast with baked french fries — Pag. 148
- **Dinner** - Mango tilapia with a side of brown rice — Pag. 101
- **Snack** - Banana walnut muffin — Pag. 48

Day 9:
- **Breakfast** - 2 eggs and 3 strips of turkey bacon — -
- **Lunch** - Avocado chicken salad sandwich — Pag. 90
- **Dinner** - Turkey and mushroom burgers on a whole wheat bun — Pag. 122
- **Snack** - Banana walnut muffin — Pag. 48

Day 10:
- **Breakfast** - Banana walnut muffin and an apple — Pag. 48
- **Lunch** - Turkey and mushroom burger on a whole wheat bun — Pag. 122
- **Dinner** - Pork chops and apples — Pag. 111
- **Snack** - Banana walnut muffin — Pag. 48

Day 11
- **Breakfast** - a bowl of oatmeal topped with peanut butter — -
- **Lunch** - Chicken breast and a Waldorf salad — Pag. 93
- **Dinner** - Kung pao chicken — Pag. 108
- **Snack** - Banana walnut muffin — Pag. 48

Day 12:
- **Breakfast** - Banana walnut muffin and a banana — Pag. 48
- **Lunch** - Lentil burgers in a wrap with a side salad — Pag. 102
- **Dinner** - Udon noodle salad with salmon — Pag. 86
- **Snack** - low fat Greek yogurt and berries — -

Day 13:
- **Breakfast** - Oatmeal with berries — -
- **Lunch** - Lentil burger on a whole wheat bun — Pag. 102
- **Dinner** - Butternut soup and a slice of wholegrain toast — Pag. 140
- **Snack** - Banana walnut muffin — Pag. 48

Day 14:
- **Breakfast** - Oatmeal with maple syrup — -
- **Lunch** - Butternut soup — Pag. 140
- **Dinner** - Turkey meatballs with low acid tomato sauce over pasta — Pag. 117 – Pag. 144
- **Snack** - An apple and banana — -

~ Week 2 Shopping List ~

Vegetables:
- ½ cup Baby Bella mushrooms
- 1 small English cucumber
- 1 red sweet pepper
- 4 stalks celery
- 2 lbs shiitake mushrooms,
- 1 head of lettuce
- ¼ cup grated carrot
- ¾ cup chopped kale
- ½ cup cilantro leaves
- 4 oz snow peas
- 2 small bunches of baby bok choy
- 3-inch piece of ginger root
- 2 potatoes
- 1 small avocado

Fruit:
- 1 bag frozen strawberries
- 5 bananas
- 1 lbs of mango chunks
- 4 medium granny smith apples
- 2 medium red delicious apple
- ¼ cup raisins

Protein:
- 8 oz skinless salmon filet
- 6 egg
- 6 chicken breast
- ¾ lbs turkey breast
- 4, 6-oz tilapia filets
- Pack of turkey bacon
- 2, 4 oz center cut pork chops

Dairy:
- small pot plain nonfat Greek yogurt
- 1 tub low-fat sour cream
- ⅓ cup grated sharp cheddar cheese

Grains:
- 2 Whole wheat burger bun
- 1 small bag dry roasted peanuts
- 1 bag jasmine rice
- 1 bag rolled oats
- ¼ cup walnuts
- 1 bag of long grain rice
- ½ cup of chopped walnuts
- 1 bag lentils
- 1 box dried bread crumbs
- 4 oz udon or buckwheat noodles
- small bag shredded coconut

Condiments:
- Worcestershire sauce
- low-fat mayonnaise
- low-sodium soy sauce
- Honey mustard dressing

Sweeteners:
- 1 bottle honey
- 1 bag of sugar
- 1 bottle vanilla extract
- 1 bottle maple syrup

Herbs and Spices:
- Garlic powder
- Onion powder
- Dried thyme
- Cumin

Liquids:
- 1 small bottle mango juice
- 1 bottle rice wine vinegar
- 1 bottle of apple cider vinegar
- 1 small bottle sweet, white wine

Oils:
- 1 bottle canola oil
- 1 bottle olive oil
- 1 bottle coconut oil
- 1 bottle sesame oil

Dry Baking Ingredients:
- 1 small bag whole wheat flour
- 1 packet baking powder
- 1 packet cornstarch

Day 15:
- **Breakfast** - Buttermilk pancakes and blueberries — Pag. 49
- **Lunch** - Turkey meatball wrap with baked french fries — Pag. 100 - Pag. 148
- **Dinner** - Seared salmon and chickpea salad — Pag. 88
- **Snack** - Turmeric ginger smoothie — Pag. 77

Day 16:
- **Breakfast** - Buttermilk pancakes and a banana — Pag. 49
- **Lunch** - Mango chicken salad — Pag. 91
- **Dinner** - Gnocchi with basil pesto — Pag. 131 – Pag. 145
- **Snack** - Air-popped popcorn — -

Day 17:
- **Breakfast** - Overnight oats — Pag. 52
- **Lunch** - Tuna salad sandwich — Pag. 94
- **Dinner** - Creamy mac and cheese — Pag. 128
- **Snack** - 1 slice of toast and peanut butter — -

Day 18:
- **Breakfast** - Granola and Yogurt — Pag. 50
- **Lunch** - Chicken breast and Caprese salad — Pag. 92
- **Dinner** - Shrimp and pea stir fry over rice noodles — Pag. 127
- **Snack** - Peanut Butter and banana shake — Pag. 78

Day 19:
- **Breakfast** - French toast — Pag. 54
- **Lunch** - Shrimp stir fry in a wrap — Pag. 127
- **Dinner** - Baked chicken thighs with a baked potato — -
- **Snack** - Air-popped popcorn — -

Day 20:
- **Breakfast** - Granola and Yogurt — Pag. 50
- **Lunch** - Spring vegetable quinoa salad — Pag. 89
- **Dinner** - Chickpea and lentil soup — Pag. 138
- **Snack** - 1 banana — -

Day 21:
- **Breakfast** - French toast — Pag. 54
- **Lunch** - Chicken breast and roast vegetables in a wrap — -
- **Dinner** - Chickpea and lentil soup with a slice of whole wheat toast — Pag. 138
- **Snack** - Strawberry banana smoothie — Pag. 67

~ Week 3 Shopping List ~

Vegetables:
- 1 large thumb of ginger
- 4 potatoes
- 2, 28-oz. cans no salt added diced tomatoes
- 4 oz dried lentils
- 4 oz celery
- 4 oz carrots
- 4 oz dried chickpeas
- 1 large packet of frozen vegetables
- 1 bunch arugula
- 3 radishes
- 1 bunch fresh basil leaves
- ½ lbs asparagus
- 1 bag frozen peas
- 1 fresh sweet bell pepper
- ⅔ lbs white cabbage
- 10 oz Yukon Gold potatoes
- 4 large ribs celery
- ½ red bell pepper, diced
- 2 large carrots
- 1 large green bell pepper
- 2 medium yellow squash
- 2, 15 oz cans no salt added chickpeas
- 1 package frozen spinach
- 2 lbs butternut squash

Fruit:
- 1 large mango
- ½ lbs fresh strawberries
- 6 bananas
- 8 fresh or canned apricot slices
- 1 packet of fresh blueberries

Protein:
- 2 lbs chicken breasts
- 4 chicken thighs
- 9 large eggs
- 2 cans of tuna in salt water
- ¾ lbs large shrimp
- 16 oz salmon filet
- 1 lbs ground turkey meat

Dairy:
- ¼ cup non-fat yogurt
- 16 oz plain nonfat Greek yogurt
- 80 oz part-skim mozzarella cheese
- 1 litre 2% milk
- 5 oz reduced-fat cheddar cheese
- 1 block unsalted butter
- 1 bottle nonfat buttermilk

Grains:
- ½ lbs quinoa
- 1 tortilla wrap
- 1 package Rice noodles
- 8 oz whole wheat penne pasta
- Popcorn seeds
- 1 loaf of whole wheat bread
- ½ lbs soft bread crumbs
- 1 oz slivered almonds
- 1 package rolled oats

Condiments:
- 1 bottle dijon mustard
- 1 jar reduced-fat mayonnaise
- 1 jar peanut butter
- 1 bottle powdered peanut butter

Sweeteners:
- 1 bottle maple syrup
- 1 small package sugar
- 1 bottle pure vanilla extract

Herbs and Spices:
- 1 oz fresh cilantro
- Dried oregano
- Ground nutmeg
- Turmeric
- Paprika
- Dried rosemary
- 3 bay leaves
- Onion powder
- Garlic powder
- 1 package fresh dill
- Dried thyme leaves

Liquids:
- 1 small bottle mango juice
- 1 bottle white wine vinegar
- 1 bottle apple cider vinegar
- 32 oz no salt added vegetable stock
- 1 small bottle coconut water
- 32 oz carrot juice

Oils:
- Olive oil
- Sesame oil

Dry Baking Ingredients:
- 1 small package all-purpose white flour
- 1 packet baking powder
- 1 packet baking soda
- 1 small packet whole wheat flour

Day 22:
- **Breakfast** - Lowfat yogurt and blueberries — -
- **Lunch** - Chicken breast and roasted vegetables — -
- **Dinner** - Black bean burgers — Pag. 103
- **Snack** - Rice cakes and peanut butter — -

Day 23:
- **Breakfast** - Blueberry smoothie — Pag. 75
- **Lunch** - Black bean burger patty on a bed of lettuce — Pag. 103
- **Dinner** - Grilled chicken breast and a side salad — -
- **Snack** - A handful of almonds and a banana — -

Day 24:
- **Breakfast** - Tropical melon smoothie — Pag. 68
- **Lunch** - 2 boiled eggs and a side salad — -
- **Dinner** - Chicken and sauteed mushrooms with a side of rice — Pag. 100
- **Snack** - Watermelon and baked water crackers — -

Day 25:
- **Breakfast** - Oatmeal topped with blueberries and peanut butter — -
- **Lunch** - Grilled chicken in a sandwich with lettuce and low fat mayonnaise — -
- **Dinner** - Cashew chicken — -
- **Snack** - Chia pudding — Pag. 165

Day 26:
- **Breakfast** - French toast — Pag. 54
- **Lunch** - Mango chicken salad — Pag. 91
- **Dinner** - Chicken parmesan — Pag. 121
- **Snack** - Green smoothie — Pag. 69

Day 27:
- **Breakfast** - Strawberry and banana smoothie — Pag. 67
- **Lunch** - Chicken parmesan on a bed of lettuce — Pag. 121
- **Dinner** - Turkey white bean soup — Pag. 139
- **Snack** - Air-popped popcorn — -

Day 28:
- **Breakfast** - Granola and Yogurt — Pag. 50
- **Lunch** - Turkey white bean soup — Pag. 139
- **Dinner** - Pecan crusted trout and rice — Pag. 119
- **Snack** - Chia pudding — Pag. 165

~ Week 4 Shopping List ~

Vegetables:
- 3, 15 oz can no salt added white beans
- 5 large ribs celery
- 3 large carrots
- 1 red bell pepper
- 1 bag frozen shelled edamame beans
- 1 tray mushrooms
- 1 lbs boneless, skinless chicken breasts
- 1 large thumb fresh ginger
- 1 cucumber
- 1 head of lettuce
- 1 bag frozen spinach
- 1 green pepper
- 2, 15 oz cans of black beans

Fruit:
- 6 oz cantaloupe
- 4 bananas
- 1 tray fresh strawberries
- 1 bag frozen mango chunks
- 1 bag frozen strawberries
- 1 large mango
- 1 honeydew melon
- ¼ of a watermelon
- 1 bag frozen blueberries

Protein:
- 6 eggs
- 2, 4 oz boneless trout filets
- 2 lbs turkey meat
- 6, 4 oz boneless, skinless chicken breasts
- 1 lb boneless skinless chicken thighs
- inch cubes

Dairy:
- 1 block unsalted butter
- 2 oz low-moisture mozzarella
- 1 oz parmesan cheese
- 1 tub non-fat yogurt
- 1 carton vanilla soy milk
- 1 carton unsweetened almond milk

Grains:
- ½ lbs almonds
- Flaxseeds
- 1 ½ oz raw pecan
- 2-4 whole wheat buns
- Rice cakes
- 1 small bag brown Rice
- Popcorn seeds
- ¼ lbs chia seeds
- 4 oz raw cashews
- 1 loaf of whole wheat bread
- Water crackers
- 1 bag Rolled Oats
- 4 oz baked tortilla chips

Condiments:
- 1 jar peanut butter
- 1 jar low fat mayonnaise
- 1 bottle gluten-free tamari sauce

Sweeteners:
- Maple syrup

Herbs and Spices:
- Ground cinnamon
- 1 small bunch fresh sage
- 1 small bunch fresh rosemary
- Smoked paprika
- Dried sage
- Dried oregano
- Dried basil
- Dried tarragon
- Dried marjoram
- 1 small package fresh dill
- Onion powder
- Garlic powder
- 1 small bunch fresh cilantro
- Ground cumin
- Ground coriander

Liquids:
- 1 small bottle mango juice
- 1 small jar low-acid tomato sauce (or home-made)
- 1 small bottle white wine
- 32 oz carton no salt added vegetable broth
- 1 small bottle apple juice

Oils:
- 1 bottle olive oil
- 1 bottle dark sesame oil

Dry Baking Ingredients:
- 1 small bag whole wheat flour
- 1 small bag of all-purpose flour

Chapter 4

Recipes

This section is filled with delicious recipes that you can make at home. There is a wide variety of meals and types of foods. You will not run out of things to cook if you try out these recipes. There is something for everyone.

The best part is that they are all acid reflux friendly. There are no specific triggers in these recipes, and they are all delicious. They have been divided into categories, so it will be easy to find what you are looking for. It is also easy to find out whether the recipes are vegan, vegetarian, or gluten-free. All you have to do is look at the tags. These specific diets have been taken into account, so there is no need to worry if you follow a stricter diet.

Eating for acid reflux does not have to be limiting and boring. There are plenty of different meals you can make. It also does not have to be hard to change your diet. Many people quit when they have to change their eating habits because it seems too hard to switch over. Most of these recipes are super easy and quick. There are a few that take a bit longer and are more technical, but you can save those for days when you want to be a little fancy or have more time.

The best strategy is to try a few new recipes each week until you find the ones you really like. It is not expected for you to be making new meals every day. But in the beginning, you will need to experiment, especially if your current diet is filled with acid reflux triggers. So jump in and find your new favorite, go-to meals.

MEASUREMENT CONVERSIONS

Volume equivalents (Liquid)

US standard	US Ounces	Metric (approximate)
2 tablespoons	1 fl. Oz.	30 mL
¼ cup	2 fl. Oz.	60 mL
½ cup	4 fl. Oz.	120 mL
1 cup	8 fl. Oz.	240 mL
1½ cup	12 fl. Oz.	355 mL
2 cups or 1 pint	16 fl. Oz.	475 mL
4 cups or 1 quart	32 fl. Oz.	1 L
1 gallon	128 fl. Oz.	4 L

Volume equivalents (Dry)

US standard	Metric (approximate)
⅛ teaspoon	0.5 mL
¼ teaspoon	1 mL
½ teaspoon	2 mL
¾ teaspoon	4 mL
1 teaspoon	5 mL
1 tablespoon	15 mL
¼ cup	59 mL
⅓ cup	79 mL
½ cup	118 mL
⅔ cup	156 mL
¾ cup	177 mL
1 cup	235 mL
2 cups or 1 pint	475 mL
3 cups	700 mL
4 cups or 1 quart	1 L

Oven Temperatures	
Fahrenheit	Celsius (approximate)
250° F	120° C
300° F	150° C
325° F	165° C
350° F	180° C
375° F	190° C
400° F	200° C
425° F	220° C
450° F	230° C

Weight Equivalents	
US Standard	Metric (approximate)
½ ounce	15 g
1 ounce	30 g
2 ounces	60 g
4 ounces	115 g
8 ounces	225 g
12 ounces	340 g
16 ounces or 1 pound	455 g

You know what they say, breakfast is the most important meal of the day. While I don't know if there is any scientific evidence for that, breakfast is a crucial meal. It will help set you up for the rest of the day and give you the energy you need in the morning.

Most people don't have the time to spend a long time preparing breakfast in the morning. Quick breakfasts are the name of the game. Most of these are super fast and easy to make, or you can make a big batch on the weekend and take a serving for breakfast every morning. Find what works for you. Just make sure you get the nutrients you need with each meal. If you feel that you need a bit more nutrients in your meals, you could add some fruit. Fruit goes with almost every breakfast food, so pick your favorite and chop on that.

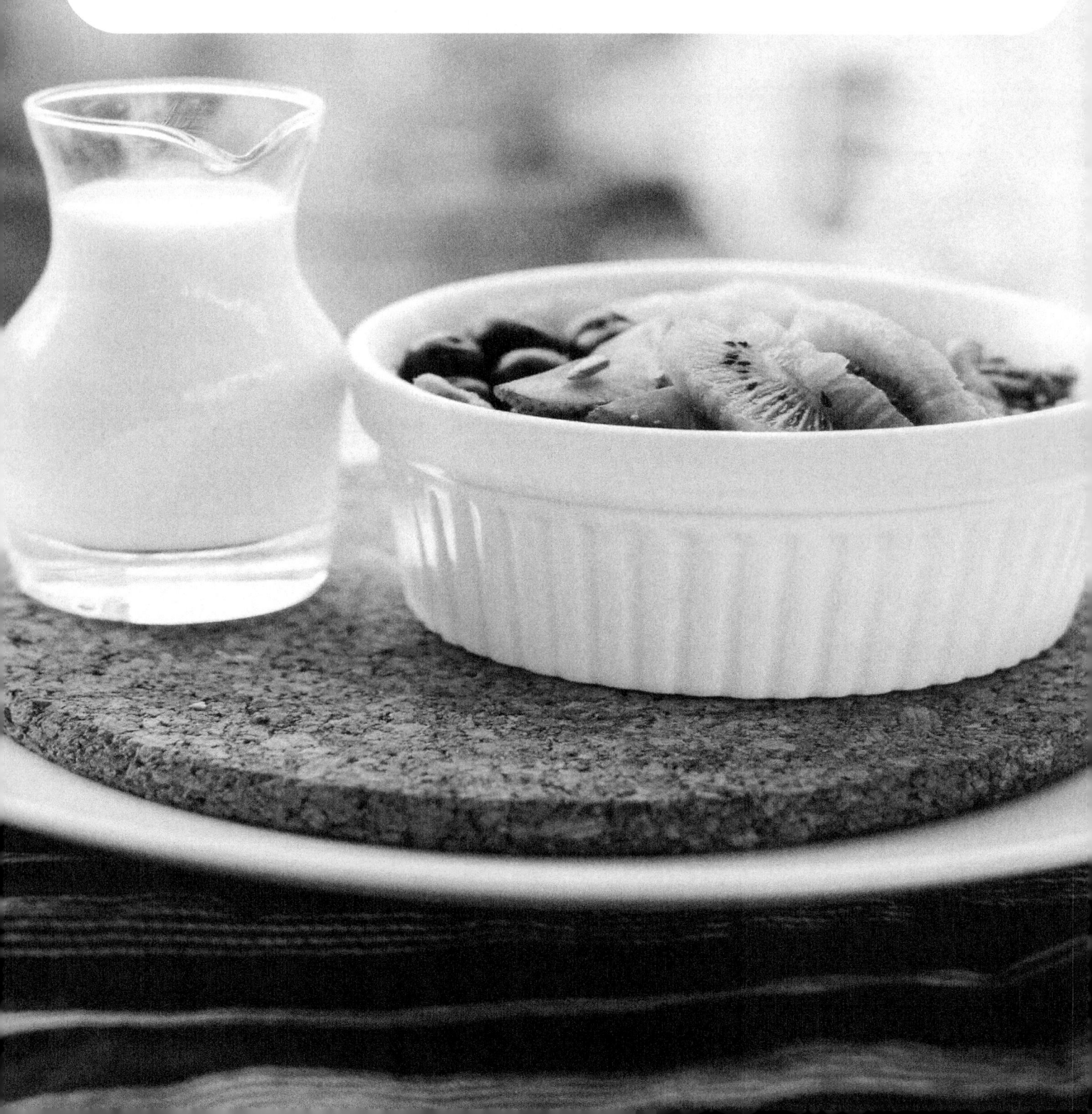

Breakfast

Banana Walnut Muffins	VEGETARIAN	48
Buttermilk Pancakes	VEGETARIAN	49
Granola	VEGETARIAN	50
Hash Browns	VEGAN	51
Overnight Oats	VEGETARIAN	52
Blueberry Muffins	VEGETARIAN	53
French Toast	VEGETARIAN	54
Roasted Vegetable Breakfast Tacos	VEGAN	55
Sweet Potato Toast With Ginger-Honey Almond Butter and Kiwi	GLUTEN-FREE VEGETARIAN	56
Simple Granola	VEGAN	57
Baked Apple Pancake	VEGETARIAN	58
Roasted Veggie and Goat Cheese Frittata	VEGETARIAN	59
Zucchini Bread	VEGETARIAN	60
Apple and Cinnamon Bread	VEGETARIAN	62

Banana Walnut Muffins

Cal 162
VEGETARIAN

Difficulty: Easy
Preparation time: 10 minutes
Cook time: 20 minutes
Servings: 18

Nutrition per serving (g)

Fat	Saturates	Carbs	Sugars	Protein
7.8	4.6	22.4	9.9	3.3

Ingredients

- 2 cups of whole wheat flour
- 1 teaspoon of salt
- 1 ½ teaspoons of baking powder
- ¾ cup of sugar
- ⅓ cup coconut oil (or any oil you choose)
- 2 eggs
- 3 very ripe bananas, mashed
- 1 teaspoon of vanilla extract
- ½ cup of chopped walnuts
- ½ cup of coconut, grated dried unsweetened

Method

1. Preheat your oven to 375 Fahrenheit and prepare your muffin tins. You can grease them or place muffin liners in them.
2. Mix the dry ingredients in a bowl.
3. Mix all the wet ingredients together, including the bananas.
4. Add the wet ingredients to the dry and combine.
5. Stir in the walnuts and coconut.
6. Pour in the batter into your muffin tin. Each case should be about ⅔ full.
7. Let the muffins bake for about 15 to 20 minutes. Insert a toothpick into them, and if it comes out clean, you know it's done.
8. Remove them from the oven and let them cool on a wire rack before serving.

These muffins freeze well. If you aren't planning on eating them all in the next few days, just pop them in the freezer. Reheat them in the microwave or let them thaw out for a few hours before eating.

Buttermilk Pancakes

Cal 360 VEGETARIAN

Difficulty: Easy
Preparation time: 10 minutes
Cook time: 20 minutes
Servings: 2 (2 pancakes per serving)

Nutrition per serving (g)

Fat	Saturates	Carbs	Sugars	Protein
13	6	50	14	12

Ingredients

- 6 tablespoons all-purpose flour
- 6 tablespoons whole wheat flour
- 1 teaspoon sugar
- 1 teaspoon baking powder
- ⅔ cup nonfat buttermilk
- 2 large eggs
- 1 teaspoon pure vanilla extract
- 2 teaspoons (per serving) unsalted butter
- 1 tablespoon (per serving) pure maple syrup

Method

1. Sift the flour, sugar, and baking powder into a bowl.
2. Whisk together the buttermilk, eggs, and vanilla extract, then add it to the dry ingredients.
3. Heat a nonstick pan on the stove.
4. Once the pan is hot enough, pour ¼ a cup of the batter into the pan.
5. Let the batter cook for about 2 minutes, until bubbles form on the surface of the batter.
6. Flip the pancake and cook until it is golden brown on the other side.
7. Once all the pancakes are done, top with butter and syrup and serve.

Granola

Cal 120 VEGETARIAN	Difficulty: Easy Preparation time: 10 minutes Cook time: 15 minutes Servings: 12

Nutrition per serving (g)

Fat	Saturates	Carbs	Sugars	Protein
4	2	20	7	2

Ingredients

- 6 cups rolled oats
- 6 cups wheat germ
- 1 cup salad oil
- 1 cup honey

Method

1. Preheat the oven to 350 degrees Fahrenheit.
2. Mix all the ingredients into a bowl, then transfer to a baking sheet.
3. Spread the mixture out and bake for 15 minutes.
4. Mix halfway through cooking.
5. Remove and let cool before serving.

Hash Browns

Cal 113

VEGAN

Difficulty: Easy
Preparation time: 15 minutes
Cook time: 15 minutes
Servings: 2

Nutrition per serving (g)

Fat	Saturates	Carbs	Sugars	Protein
4	2	18	1	2

Ingredients

- 8 oz of potatoes, shredded (Yukon Gold potatoes work best)
- ⅛ teaspoons salt
- 2 teaspoons unsalted butter

Method

1. Shred your potatoes using a grater.
2. Place the shredded potatoes into a strainer and press down on them with a spatula. Get as much water out as possible.
3. Place them on two layers of paper towels and pat them dry. Try and get them as dry as possible.
4. Once dry, put them in a bowl. Sprinkle with salt and mix.
5. Heat up a pan on the stove and add butter.
6. Once the butter is bubbling, add the potatoes. Toss them around in the pan for about 5 minutes so that they can cook evenly.
7. Once this is done, create two piles of potatoes in the pan.
8. Press them down and make them flat. If the heat is too hot, you can lower it to a medium temperature.
9. Let it cook for about 5 minutes, making sure it doesn't burn. It should be a golden-brown color.
10. Flip it and let it cook on the other side for about 5 minutes.
11. Once both sides are crispy and golden, serve immediately.

Overnight Oats

Cal **279** VEGETARIAN	**Difficulty:** Easy **Preparation time:** 5 minutes **Cook time:** 0 minutes **Servings:** 1

Nutrition per serving (g)

Fat	Saturates	Carbs	Sugars	Protein
3	1	48	19	17

Ingredients

- ½ cup skim milk or vanilla almond milk
- ¼ cup plain nonfat Greek yogurt
- 1 teaspoon honey
- 1 teaspoon vanilla
- ½ cup rolled oats
- ½ cup any fruit

Method

1. Place all the ingredients into a jar with a lid.
2. Mix until well combined.
3. Leave in the fridge overnight and then serve the next day.

Blueberry Muffins

Cal 163 VEGETARIAN

Difficulty: Normal
Preparation time: 15 minutes
Cook time: 15 minutes
Servings: 6

Nutrition per serving (g)

Fat	Saturates	Carbs	Sugars	Protein
3	1	2	3	6

Ingredients

- 2 teaspoons of canola oil
- ½ cup sweetener of choice
- 1 large egg
- 2 tablespoons of nonfat yogurt
- ½ teaspoon of pure vanilla extract
- 1 cup all-purpose white flour
- ½ cup whole wheat flour
- 2 tablespoons wheat germ
- ¼ teaspoon salt
- 1 teaspoon baking powder
- ¼ teaspoon baking soda
- ½ cup low-fat buttermilk
- ½ cup blueberries

Method

1. Preheat your oven to 375 degrees Fahrenheit.
2. Crack your eggs and separate the egg whites and egg yolks into separate bowls. Set the yolks aside.
3. Whisk the whites until they turn frothy.
4. In a separate bowl, cream the egg yolk, vanilla extract, yogurt, oil, and sweetener.
5. Sift the flour, wheat germ, baking powder, baking soda, and salt in the creamed mixture.
6. Fold together both mixtures.
7. Add the buttermilk until the mixture is smooth. Be careful not to overmix.
8. Fold in the frothed up egg whites. Then fold in the blueberries.
9. Pour the batter into a lined muffin tin.
10. Bake for 12 to 15 minutes or until a toothpick comes out clean.

French Toast

Cal **290** VEGETARIAN	**Difficulty:** Easy **Preparation time:** 5 minutes **Cook time:** 20 minutes **Servings:** 2 (2 slices per serving)

Nutrition per serving (g)

Fat	Saturates	Carbs	Sugars	Protein
8	2.5	42	15	8

Ingredients

- 2 large eggs
- 1 teaspoon sugar
- 6 tablespoons 2% milk (or milk of choice)
- ¼ teaspoon ground nutmeg
- ½ teaspoon pure vanilla extract
- 3 teaspoon unsalted butter
- 4, 1 oz slices of sourdough bread
- 2 tablespoons pure maple syrup

Method

1. Whisk the eggs, milk, sugar, nutmeg, and vanilla in a bowl.
2. Place a nonstick pan on the stove to heat up.
3. Place a slice of bread into the mixture, and when it is well-coated, place it in the pan.
4. Let it cook for 3 to 4 minutes on each side. They should be golden and crispy on the outside.
5. Repeat this with the remaining bread.
6. Serve by topping with the butter and maple syrup.

Roasted Vegetable Breakfast Tacos

Cal 297 — VEGAN

Difficulty: Easy
Preparation time: 10 minutes
Cook time: 15 minutes
Servings: 2

Nutrition per serving (g)

Fat	Saturates	Carbs	Sugars	Protein
8	1	48	5	10

Ingredients

- 1 small sweet potato, cubed
- 1 medium carrot, peeled and sliced
- 1 tablespoon olive oil
- 1 teaspoon ground cumin
- ½ teaspoon ground coriander
- ¼ teaspoon salt
- 1 cup canned black beans, mashed
- 2 (6-inch) corn tortillas

Method

1. Preheat your oven to 350 degrees Fahrenheit.
2. Line a baking sheet with parchment paper.
3. Mix the sweet potatoes, carrots, olive oil, cumin, coriander, and salt together.
4. Spread them across the baking sheet and roast for 15 minutes.
5. Remove from the oven and set aside.
6. Warm up the tortilla for about 10 seconds in the microwave or quickly in a pan. Spread the mashed black beans over the tortilla.
7. Evenly distribute the roast vegetables between the two tacos.
8. Serve with a drizzle of your favorite sauce.

Sweet Potato Toast With Ginger-Honey Almond Butter and Kiwi

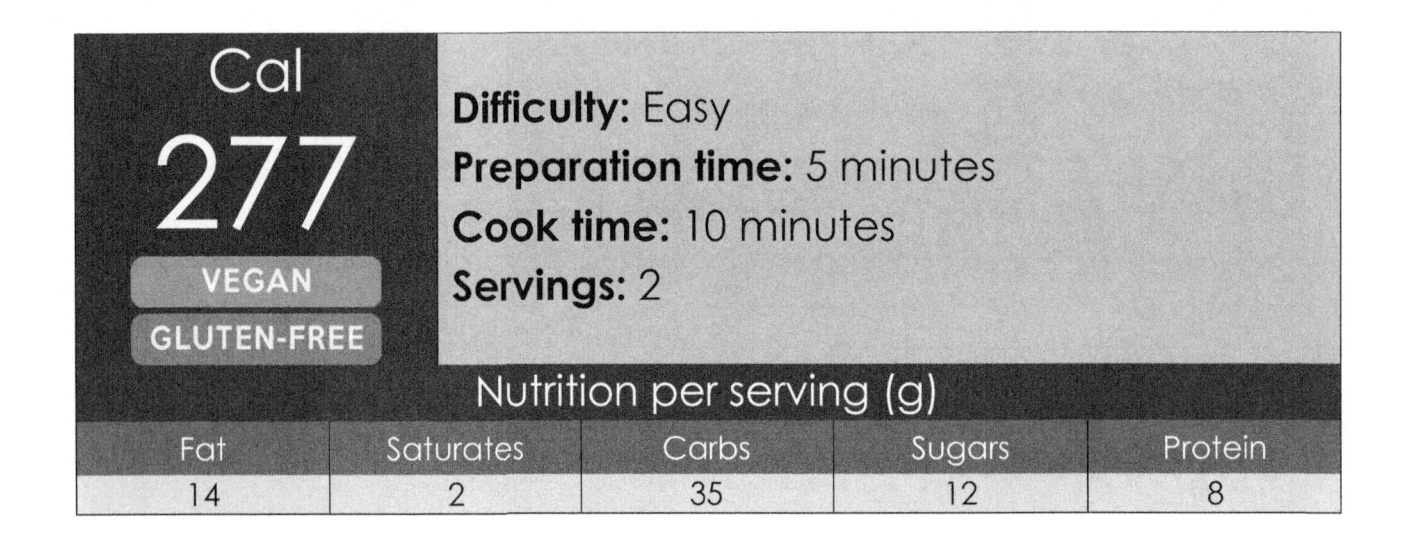

Cal 277

VEGAN
GLUTEN-FREE

Difficulty: Easy
Preparation time: 5 minutes
Cook time: 10 minutes
Servings: 2

Nutrition per serving (g)

Fat	Saturates	Carbs	Sugars	Protein
14	2	35	12	8

Ingredients

- 1 medium sweet potato, peeled or unpeeled
- 3 tablespoons almond butter
- ½ teaspoon honey
- ¼ teaspoon ground ginger
- 2 medium kiwi, peeled or unpeeled

Method

1. Slice the sweet potato, lengthways, into ¼ inch slices.
2. Stir the almond butter, ginger, and honey, in a small bowl until combined.
3. Place the sweet potato slices in a toaster and toast until thoroughly cooked through. This might take two or three toasting sessions.
4. Once cooked through, leave it on one side to cool down for a minute or so.
5. Spread the almond butter mixture over the sweet potato and top it with kiwi slices.
6. You can add any extra topping you would like to this dish. Serve.

Simple Granola

Cal 239 — VEGAN

Difficulty: Normal
Preparation time: 10 minutes
Cook time: 45 minutes
Servings: 6

Nutrition per serving (g)

Fat	Saturates	Carbs	Sugars	Protein
7	1	39	10	8

Ingredients

- 3 quarts water
- 1 ⅓ cups steel cut oats
- ⅔ cup quinoa
- ¼ cup sliced almonds
- ¼ cup chopped walnuts
- ½ cup unsweetened applesauce
- ½ teaspoon ground cinnamon
- ½ teaspoon ground nutmeg
- ⅛ teaspoon salt
- 2 tablespoon pure maple syrup
- ¼ cup raisins
- ¼ cup dried cranberries

Method

1. Preheat your oven to 300 degrees Fahrenheit.
2. Place a small pot of water on to boil and pour in the oats and quinoa.
3. Reduce the heat to a simmer and allow the oats and quinoa to cook for 12 minutes.
4. Drain and rinse the oats and quinoa with cold water to stop them from cooking any longer.
5. Place them in a large bowl with the rest of the ingredients. Toss until everything is mixed together.
6. Line a baking sheet with aluminum foil.
7. Pour the granola on the sheet and spread out as much as possible.
8. Allow baking in the oven for 45 minutes. Stir every 15 minutes or so.
9. Remove from the oven and let it cool.
10. Store in an airtight container and enjoy with fresh fruit, yogurt, or milk.

Baked Apple Pancake

Cal 201 — VEGETARIAN

Difficulty: Normal
Preparation time: 10 minutes
Cook time: 35 minutes
Servings: 4

Nutrition per serving (g)

Fat	Saturates	Carbs	Sugars	Protein
6	3	39	11	8

Ingredients

- 4 medium apples
- 2 teaspoons unsalted butter
- ½ cup sugar
- ¼ cup water
- 3 large egg whites
- 1 large egg yolk
- ¾ cup nonfat buttermilk
- ¾ cup all-purpose white flour
- ¼ teaspoon salt
- 2 tablespoons sugar
- 2 teaspoons unsalted butter

Method

1. Peel the apples and remove the cores, then thinly slice.
2. Preheat the oven to 425 degrees Fahrenheit.
3. Heat up the butter in a nonstick skillet.
4. Pour in the sugar and water and let it boil.
5. Place the apples in the pan and let it cook for about 15 minutes.
6. Stir the apples every few minutes.
7. As it cooks, the liquid should start browning, and the bottom of the apples should turn the same color.
8. Take out your blender or food processor and pour in the egg whites, egg yolk, buttermilk, flour, salt, and the two tablespoons of sugar. Blend together.
9. Once the apples are done cooking, pour over this mixture. The liquid should cover all the apples.
10. Transfer the skillet to the oven and bake for 15 to 18 minutes.
11. Once the pancake is brown on the top and cooked through the middle, it can be removed from the oven.
12. Put two teaspoons of butter over the top and let it melt; Cut it into four pieces and serve.

Roasted Veggie and Goat Cheese Frittata

Cal 110 VEGETARIAN

Difficulty: Normal
Preparation time: 10 minutes
Cook time: 30 minutes
Servings: 6

Nutrition per serving (g)

Fat	Saturates	Carbs	Sugars	Protein
7	3	5	2	7

Ingredients

- ½ medium zucchini, diced into medium pieces
- ½ cup small broccoli florets
- 1 medium carrot, diced into small pieces
- ½ small sweet potato, diced into small pieces
- ½ cup Baby Bella mushrooms, sliced
- 1 teaspoon basil
- ½ teaspoon thyme
- 1 teaspoon oregano
- ¼ teaspoon salt
- 1 tablespoon olive oil
- 4 large eggs
- ⅛ teaspoon turmeric
- ¼ cup goat cheese, crumbled

Method

1. Preheat the oven to 350 degrees Fahrenheit.
2. Grease a 9-inch cake pan.
3. Pour in the vegetables along with the basil, thyme, oregano, salt, and olive oil.
4. Place in the oven and roast for about 20 minutes or until the sweet potato and carrots are soft.
5. While that is cooking, whisk the eggs, turmeric, and goat cheese.
6. Once the veggies have finished cooking, remove them from the oven and pour over the egg mixture.
7. Mix it together so that the vegetables are evenly distributed throughout the pan.
8. Place it in the oven to bake until the eggs have set. This should only take another 5 or 10 minutes.
9. Remove from the oven and allow to cool for about 5 minutes before cutting and serving.

Zucchini Bread

Cal 218 VEGETARIAN

Difficulty: Normal
Preparation time: 20 minutes
Cook time: 60 minutes
Servings: 8

Nutrition per serving (g)

Fat	Saturates	Carbs	Sugars	Protein
5	1	35	7	10

Ingredients

- ¼ cup dried pumpkin seeds
- 2 teaspoons light brown sugar
- ¼ teaspoon ground cinnamon
- 1 large egg yolk
- 1 teaspoon canola oil
- ⅔ cup sugar
- 2 tablespoons nonfat yogurt
- ½ teaspoon pure vanilla extract
- 3 large egg whites
- 1 ¼ cup all-purpose white flour
- ¾ cup whole wheat flour
- ¼ teaspoon salt
- 2 teaspoons baking powder
- ½ teaspoon baking soda
- ½ teaspoon ground cinnamon
- ¼ teaspoon ground nutmeg
- ¼ teaspoon ground cloves
- ¼ cup oatmeal (quick, not instant)
- ½ cup nonfat buttermilk
- 2 cups zucchini (grated)
- ¼ cup raisins

Method

1. Preheat your oven to 350 degrees Fahrenheit.

2. Line a bread tin with parchment paper or nonstick foil.

3. Place a skillet over high heat and pour in the pumpkin seeds. Cook until they have turned brown. If they begin to pop in the pan, take it off the heat and finish cooking in the pan.

4. Pour the seeds into a bowl with half of the sugar and half of the cinnamon. Stir it all together. Set this aside to use later.

5. Whisk the egg yolk and canola oil together until smooth.

6. Add in the remaining sugar, yogurt, and vanilla extract. Whisk together.

7. In another bowl, whisk the egg whites until frothy. Do not whisk until stiff peaks are formed. This means you have whisked too much.

8. Sift the flour, whole wheat flour, salt, baking powder, baking soda, cinnamon, nutmeg, and cloves into a bowl.

9. Pour in the oats.

10. Add the egg yolk mixture and fold this together.

11. Mix in the zucchini and raisins.

12. Pour in the buttermilk and combine until smooth.

13. Pour the batter into the prepared bread tin.

14. Sprinkle over the pumpkin seed mixture and bake for 60 minutes.

15. The bread is ready when you pierce the middle with a toothpick, and it comes out clean.

16. Remove from the oven and allow to cool.

17. Cut into slices and serve. Keep fresh in an airtight container.

Apple and Cinnamon Bread

Cal 196 — VEGETARIAN

Difficulty: Normal
Preparation time: 20 minutes
Cook time: 60 minutes
Servings: 8

Nutrition per serving (g)

Fat	Saturates	Carbs	Sugars	Protein
5	1	33	6	7

Ingredients

- ¼ cup pecans, coarsely chopped
- 2 teaspoons maple syrup
- ¼ teaspoon ground cinnamon
- 1 large egg yolk
- 1 teaspoon canola oil
- ⅔ cup sugar
- ½ cup unsweetened applesauce
- ½ teaspoon pure vanilla extract
- 3 large egg whites
- 1 ¼ cups all-purpose white flour
- ¾ cup whole wheat flour
- ¼ teaspoon salt
- 2 teaspoons baking powder
- ½ teaspoon baking soda
- 1 teaspoon ground cinnamon
- ¼ cup wheat germ
- 2 cups apples, peeled and grated
- ½ cup low-fat buttermilk

Method

1. Preheat the oven to 350 degrees Fahrenheit.

2. Line a bread tin with parchment paper or nonstick foil.

3. Stir together the pecans, maple syrup, and cinnamon. Set it aside.

4. Whisk the egg yolk and canola oil together until smooth.

5. Add in the remaining sugar, apple sauce, and vanilla extract. Whisk together.

6. In another bowl, whisk the egg whites until frothy. Do not whisk until stiff peaks are formed. This means you have whisked too much.

7. Sift the flour, whole wheat flour, salt, baking powder, baking soda, cinnamon, and wheat germ into a bowl.

8. Fold in the egg yolk mixture, then add the apples.

9. Pour in the buttermilk and mix together until the batter is smooth.

10. Fold in the egg whites.

11. Pour the batter into the baking pan.

12. Take the pecan mixture and spread it out on top of the batter.

13. Bake for 60 minutes.

14. The bread is ready when you pierce the middle with a toothpick, and it comes out clean.

15. Remove from the oven and allow to cool.

16. Cut into slices and serve. Keep fresh in an airtight container.

Smoothies are extremely easy to make, delicious, and filling. It is also a great way to get some extra servings of fruit and even vegetables into your diet. All you need is a good blender. If you don't have a blender, I would highly suggest investing in one. You can use them for so many things, including making delicious smoothies.

You can play around with ingredients and ratios until you find something you really love. Smoothies can be used as a quick on-the-go breakfast or just a yummy snack in the middle of the day. It is a cold drink that makes it perfect for summer. If you add some extra ice and lower the amount of liquid in these recipes, you can make thicker smoothies and smoothie bowls. These have the consistency of ice-cream or sorbet. You can top these with whatever you want. It is a great way to start the day or to have a healthy dessert.

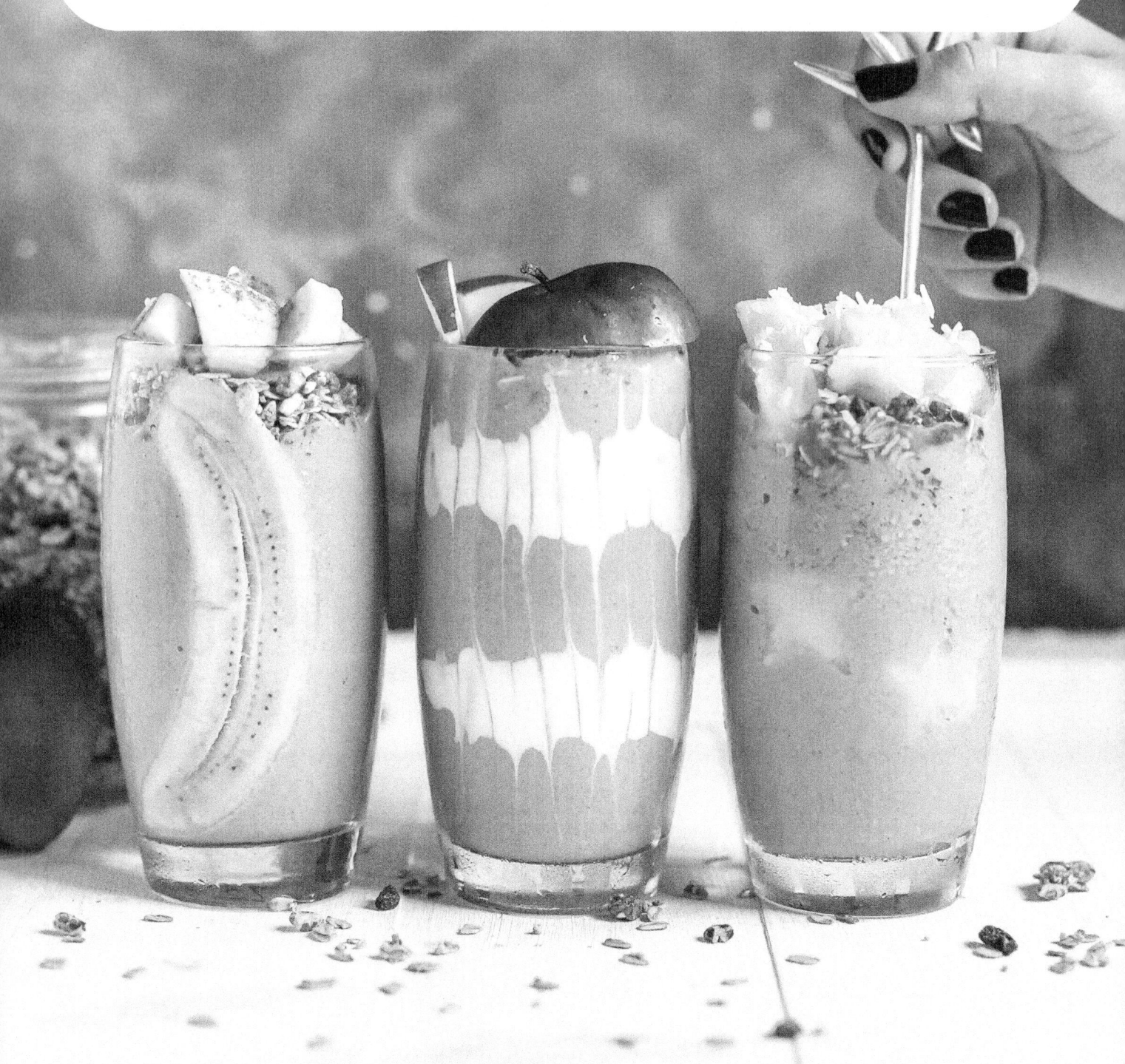

Smoothie

Sweet Pea Smoothie	VEGAN	GLUTEN-FREE	66
Strawberry Banana Smoothie	VEGETARIAN	GLUTEN-FREE	67
Tropical Melon Smoothie	VEGETARIAN	GLUTEN-FREE	68
Green Smoothie	VEGAN	GLUTEN-FREE	69
Kale and Ginger Smoothie	VEGAN	GLUTEN-FREE	70
Spinach, Mango, and Melon Smo…	VEGAN	GLUTEN-FREE	71
Alkaline Smoothie	VEGAN	GLUTEN-FREE	72
Melon Smoothie	VEGAN	GLUTEN-FREE	73
Apple Smoothie with Wheatgerm	VEGETARIAN		74
Blueberry Smoothie	VEGAN	GLUTEN-FREE	75
Almond Milk Smoothie	VEGETARIAN	GLUTEN-FREE	76
Turmeric Ginger Smoothie	VEGETARIAN	GLUTEN-FREE	77
Peanut Butter and Banana Shake	VEGETARIAN	GLUTEN-FREE	78

Sweet Pea Smoothie

Cal 190

VEGAN
GLUTEN-FREE

Difficulty: Easy
Preparation time: 5 minutes
Cook time: 0 minutes
Servings: 2

Nutrition per serving (g)

Fat	Saturates	Carbs	Sugars	Protein
0	0	43	26	3

Ingredients

- 1 1/2 cup mango juice
- 1 cup frozen strawberries
- 1/3 cup frozen peas
- 1 banana

Method

1. Cook the peas for 5 minutes in boiling water. Drain and cool.
2. Add all the ingredients to a blender and blend until smooth.
3. Serve.

Strawberry Banana Smoothie

Cal 234

VEGETARIAN
GLUTEN-FREE

Difficulty: Easy
Preparation time: 5 minutes
Cook time: 0 minutes
Servings: 1

Nutrition per serving (g)

Fat	Saturates	Carbs	Sugars	Protein
1	0	51	40	9

Ingredients

- ¼ cup non-fat yogurt
- 1 cup fresh strawberries
- ½ cup mango juice
- ½ banana

Method

1. Place all the ingredients into a blender and blend on high.
2. Once it is all smooth, pour into a glass, and serve.

Tropical Melon Smoothie

Cal 215

VEGETARIAN
GLUTEN-FREE

Difficulty: Easy
Preparation time: 5 minutes
Cook time: 0 minutes
Servings: 1

Nutrition per serving (g)

Fat	Saturates	Carbs	Sugars	Protein
1	0	47	39	9

Ingredients

- ½ cup nonfat yogurt
- 6 oz cantaloupe
- ½ banana
- ⅓ cup mango or papaya juice

Method

1. Place all the ingredients in a blender and blend on high.
2. Once smooth, pour into a glass and serve.

Green Smoothie

Cal 122	Difficulty: Easy
VEGAN **GLUTEN-FREE**	Preparation time: 5 minutes Cook time: 0 minutes Servings: 2

Nutrition per serving (g)

Fat	Saturates	Carbs	Sugars	Protein
2	0.1	27	18	2

Ingredients

- 1 cup unsweetened almond milk
- 1 cup mango chunks, frozen
- ½ cup strawberries, frozen
- 1 banana
- 1 cup spinach
- 1 teaspoon flaxseeds

Method

Add all ingredients to a blender and blend until smooth. Serve.

Kale and Ginger Smoothie

Cal 172

VEGAN
GLUTEN-FREE

Difficulty: Easy
Preparation time: 5 minutes
Cook time: 0 minutes
Servings: 2

Nutrition per serving (g)

Fat	Saturates	Carbs	Sugars	Protein
3	0	36	20	3.5

Ingredients

- 1 cup kale, cut into chunks
- 1 cup mango chunks, frozen
- 1 banana
- 1 cup cantaloupe melon, cut into chunks
- ½ inch fresh ginger, peeled
- 1 ½ cups unsweetened almond milk

Method

Place all ingredients in a blender and blend until smooth. Serve.

Spinach, Mango, and Melon Smoothie

Cal 98

VEGAN
GLUTEN-FREE

Difficulty: Easy
Preparation time: 5 minutes
Cook time: 0 minutes
Servings: 2

Nutrition per serving (g)

Fat	Saturates	Carbs	Sugars	Protein
0.4	0	25	18	1.5

Ingredients

- 1 cup spinach
- 1 cup of water
- ½ cup mango chunks, frozen
- 1 cup melon chunks, frozen
- 1 banana

Method

1. Place all the ingredients into the blender and blend until smooth.
2. Serve cold.

Alkaline Smoothie

Cal 138

VEGAN
GLUTEN-FREE

Difficulty: Easy
Preparation time: 5 minutes
Cook time: 0 minutes
Servings: 2

Nutrition per serving (g)

Fat	Saturates	Carbs	Sugars	Protein
2	0	29	21	3

Ingredients

- 1 ½ cups unsweetened almond milk
- ½ small beet, boiled
- 1 cup cherries, frozen or fresh
- 1 banana
- ½ cup spinach (optional)

Method

1. Add all the ingredients into a blender and blend until smooth.
2. Serve cold.

Melon Smoothie

Cal 167

VEGAN
GLUTEN-FREE

Difficulty: Easy
Preparation time: 5 minutes
Cook time: 0 minutes
Servings: 2

Nutrition per serving (g)

Fat	Saturates	Carbs	Sugars	Protein
4	0.4	34	23	3

Ingredients

- 1 ½ cups unsweetened almond milk
- 1 banana
- 1 cup mango chunks, frozen
- 1 cup melon chunks, frozen
- 1 tablespoon chia seeds

Method

1. Add all the ingredients to the blender and blend until smooth.
2. Serve cold.

Apple Smoothie with Wheatgerm

Cal 179
VEGETARIAN

Difficulty: Easy
Preparation time: 5 minutes
Cook time: 0 minutes
Servings: 2

Nutrition per serving (g)

Fat	Saturates	Carbs	Sugars	Protein
3	1	30	19	5

Ingredients

- 2 tablespoons Wheatgerm
- 1 large ripe banana
- ½ cup plain yogurt
- 1 tablespoon flax seeds
- 1 cup apple juice
- ¼ cup water

Method

1. Place all the ingredients into a blender and blend until smooth.
2. Serve cold.

Blueberry Smoothie

Cal 185

VEGAN
GLUTEN-FREE

Difficulty: Easy
Preparation time: 5 minutes
Cook time: 0 minutes
Servings: 2

Nutrition per serving (g)

Fat	Saturates	Carbs	Sugars	Protein
4	1	31	27	6

Ingredients

- ½ cup frozen blueberries
- ½ cup chilled apple juice
- ½ cup rolled oats
- ⅓ teaspoon ground cinnamon
- 1 cup cold almond milk

Method

1. Place all the ingredients into the blender and blend until smooth.
2. Serve cold.

Almond Milk Smoothie

Cal 144

VEGETARIAN
GLUTEN-FREE

Difficulty: Easy
Preparation time: 5 minutes
Cook time: 0 minutes
Servings: 2

Nutrition per serving (g)

Fat	Saturates	Carbs	Sugars	Protein
2	0	26	21.5	7

Ingredients

- 1 cup almond milk
- 1 cup apple juice
- ½ cup Greek yogurt (vanilla flavored)
- 6 large frozen strawberries
- ½ cup frozen mango
- 1 teaspoon turmeric

Method

1. Place all the ingredients into a blender and blend until smooth.
2. Serve cold.

Turmeric Ginger Smoothie

Cal 114

VEGETARIAN
GLUTEN-FREE

Difficulty: Easy
Preparation time: 5 minutes
Cook time: 0 minutes
Servings: 2

Nutrition per serving (g)

Fat	Saturates	Carbs	Sugars	Protein
0	0	27	21	3

Ingredients

- 2 cups chilled carrot juice
- 1 medium ripe banana
- 6 large frozen strawberries
- 1 small yogurt (4 oz.)
- 1 teaspoon turmeric
- ½ teaspoon ginger

Method

1. Place all the ingredients into a blender and blend until smooth.
2. Serve chilled.

Peanut Butter and Banana Shake

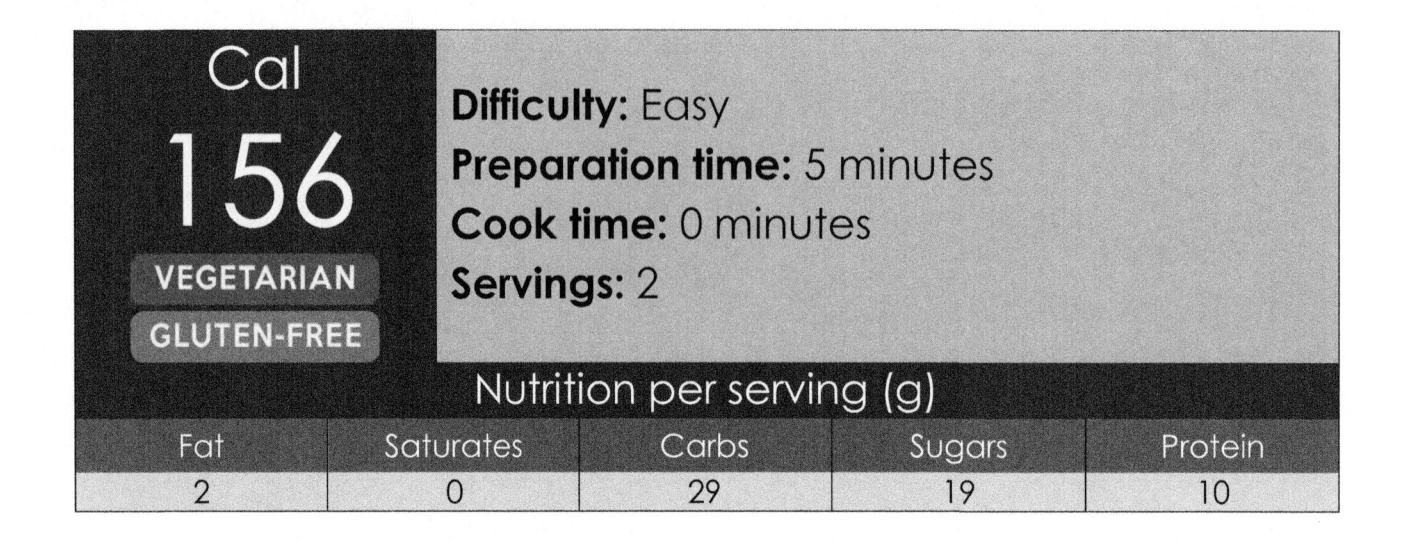

Cal 156

VEGETARIAN
GLUTEN-FREE

Difficulty: Easy
Preparation time: 5 minutes
Cook time: 0 minutes
Servings: 2

Nutrition per serving (g)

Fat	Saturates	Carbs	Sugars	Protein
2	0	29	19	10

Ingredients

- 1 medium banana, frozen and chopped
- 1 cup coconut water
- 4 oz plain nonfat Greek yogurt
- 2 tablespoons powdered peanut butter

Method

1. Place all the ingredients into a blender. The frozen banana should go first.
2. Blend until it is smooth. Serve.

Salads are a delicious low-calorie meal. Sometimes they get a bad rep for being boring and not filling. This only if you don't do it right. Obviously, if you have a big bowl of lettuce, then you will not be filled up, and it will taste bland. A salad is not about having a big bowl of leafy greens and some dressing. They can be more complex than that.

You can basically add any vegetable, protein, or grain to a salad. Having a right balance is what will make it delicious and filling. It is all about what you put in and how you cook it. Another great thing about salads is that you can add any leftovers to make a delicious lunch. It is a great way to use any leftovers in a fresh way. Take a look at these great salads and find some inspiration for your next healthy lunch.

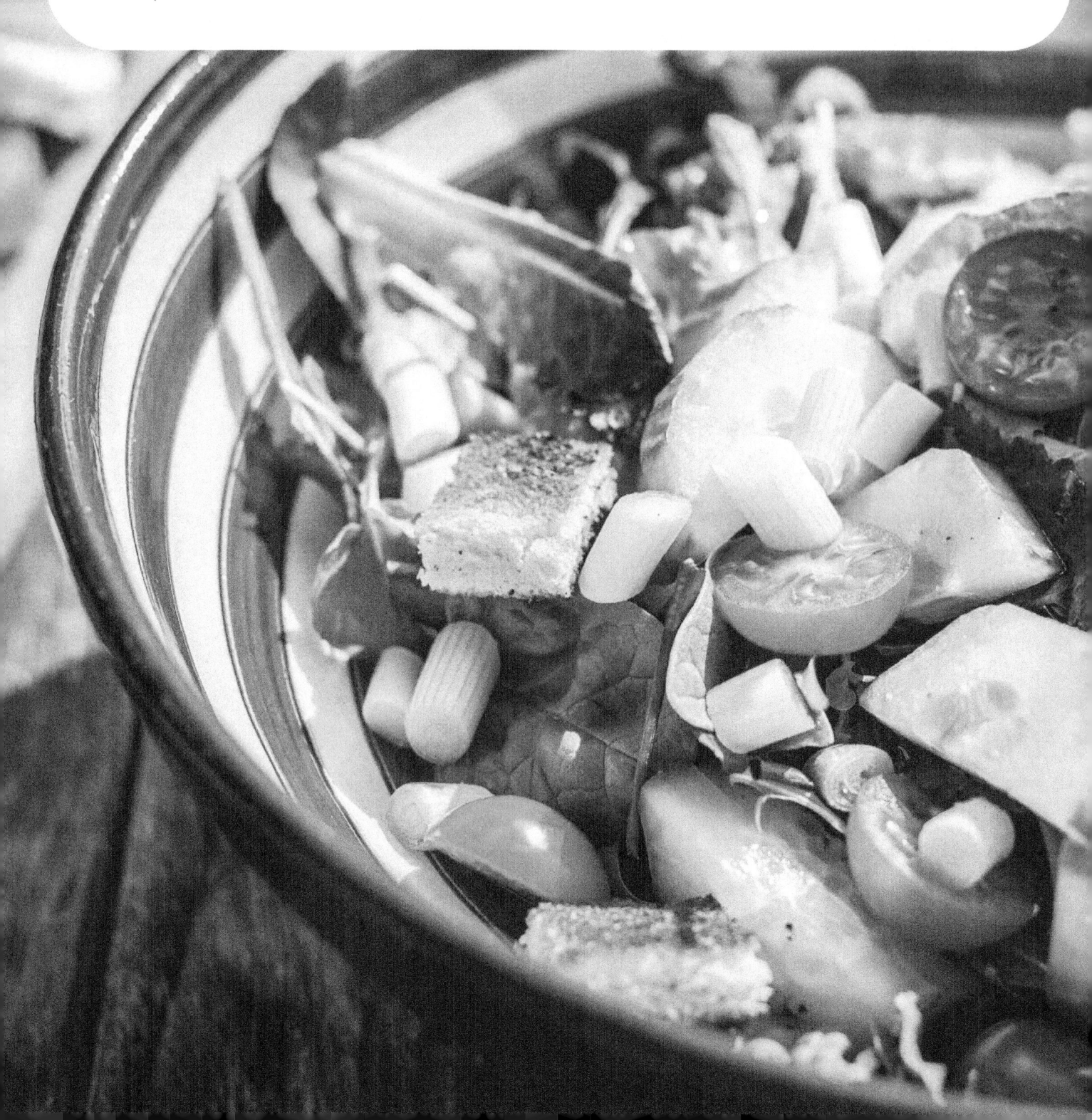

Salads

Asparagus and Green Bean Salad	GLUTEN-FREE	82
Iceberg Wedge Salad with Blue…	VEGETARIAN GLUTEN-FREE	83
Chinese Chicken Salad		84
Udon Noodle Salad with Salmon		86
Seared Salmon and Chickpea Salad	GLUTEN-FREE	88
Spring Vegetable Quinoa Salad	VEGAN	89
Light Avocado Chicken Salad		90
Mango Chicken Salad	GLUTEN-FREE	91
Apricot Caprese Salad	VEGETARIAN GLUTEN-FREE	92
Waldorf Salad	VEGETARIAN GLUTEN-FREE	93
Tuna Potato Salad	GLUTEN-FREE	94

Asparagus and Green Bean Salad

Cal 123 GLUTEN-FREE

Difficulty: Easy
Preparation time: 15 minutes
Cook time: 5 minutes
Servings: 12

Nutrition per serving (g)

Fat	Saturates	Carbs	Sugars	Protein
5.8	1.2	11.6	0.8	5.7

Ingredients

- 1 pound of fresh asparagus
- 1 pound of green beans, stems removed
- 2 tablespoons of shredded carrots
- 3 or 4 slices turkey bacon, cooked and crumbled*
- 3 hard-boiled eggs, quartered
- 2 teaspoons of Dijon mustard
- 4 teaspoons of balsamic vinegar
- 3 tablespoons of olive oil
- Salt

Method

1. Bring a pot of salted water to boil and add the asparagus and green beans. Let them cook for about 4 to 5 minutes or until tender. They should still have a crunch to them.
2. Once cooked, drain and run under cold water to stop them from cooking any farther. Place in the fridge to cool down.
3. Make a vinaigrette by mixing together the mustard, vinegar, olive oil, and salt.
4. Chop up the cooled asparagus and green beans.
5. Place them in a bowl with the carrots and turkey bacon.
6. Drizzle the vinaigrette over and toss.
7. Plate it up and add the eggs over the top. Serve.

This is optional. If you would like to make this dish vegan, you can just remove the turkey bacon. Feel free to replace it with a meat alternative like crispy tofu.

Iceberg Wedge Salad with Blue Cheese Dressing

Cal 75
GLUTEN-FREE

Difficulty: Easy
Preparation time: 5 minutes
Cook time: 0 minutes
Servings: 1

Nutrition per serving (g)

Fat	Saturates	Carbs	Sugars	Protein
3	2	9	6	4

Ingredients

- ⅛ medium head iceberg lettuce
- 1 tablespoon candied pecans
- 2 tablespoons blue cheese dressing

Method

1. Place the washed lettuce on a plate.
2. Drizzle over the dressing and sprinkle over the pecans.
3. Serve.

Chinese Chicken Salad

Cal 524	**Difficulty:** Normal **Preparation time:** 20 minutes **Cook time:** 20 minutes **Servings:** 4

Nutrition per serving (g)

Fat	Saturates	Carbs	Sugars	Protein
9	1	75.5	8.5	40.5

Ingredients

- 3 quarts water
- 8 oz whole wheat udon noodles
- 2 teaspoons dark sesame oil
- 4 oz shiitake mushrooms, thinly sliced
- Spray oil
- ¼ cup slivered almonds
- 16 oz boneless, skinless, chicken breast
- 1 tablespoon low-sodium soy sauce
- 8 oz napa cabbage, thinly sliced
- 8 oz carrots, peeled and thinly sliced
- 4 oz snow peas
- 3 tablespoons hoisin sauce
- 2 tablespoons rice vinegar
- 2 tablespoons mango juice
- 2 teaspoons black sesame seeds

Method

1. Preheat the oven to 375 degrees Fahrenheit and place a skillet inside.
2. Pour the water into a pot and place it on high heat.
3. Place the noodles into the boiling water and cook for about 6 to 8 minutes.
4. Once cooked, drain and place in a bowl with the sesame oil. Toss it and put it in the fridge for now.
5. While the noodles are cooking, place a skillet over medium heat and spray with oil.
6. Add in the mushrooms and let them cook down.
7. Once they are lightly brown, add in the almonds. Let these cook until the almonds turn golden.
8. Take them off the heat and set them aside.
9. Take out the skillet that you placed in the oven in step one and spray with oil.
10. Add the chicken and cook in the oven for 8 minutes.
11. Remove from the oven, flip the chicken, and add the soy sauce. Place back in the oven for another 5 to 8 minutes.
12. Once the chicken is cooked, remove from the oven. Cut the chicken into thin strips and leave to cool. This dish is best served cold, so place the chicken in the fridge once it has reached room temperature.
13. Make the dressing by mixing the hoisin sauce and rice vinegar. Place it in the fridge.
14. Once all the ingredients have cooked and cooled, it is time to assemble the salad. Get all of your ingredients out.
15. Toss the udon noodles, napa cabbage, carrots, snow peas, and dressing together in a large bowl.
16. Serve by topping with the mushroom and almond mixture, and the sesame seeds.

Udon Noodle Salad with Salmon

Cal 540

Difficulty: Normal
Preparation time: 15 minutes
Cook time: 45 minutes
Servings: 2

Nutrition per serving (g)

Fat	Saturates	Carbs	Sugars	Protein
16	3	61	11	41

Ingredients

- 1 tablespoon fresh ginger, minced
- ¼ garlic powder
- 1 tablespoon dark sesame oil
- 1 teaspoon rice wine vinegar
- 1 teaspoon honey
- 2 tablespoons low-sodium soy sauce
- ½ cup cilantro leaves
- 4 quarts water
- Spray oil
- 2 lbs shiitake mushrooms, cut stems off, and slice the caps
- 4 oz snow peas, stems trimmed
- 4 oz udon or buckwheat noodles
- 8 oz skinless salmon filet
- 2 small bunches of baby bok choy, sliced crosswise

Method

1. Preheat the oven to 400 degrees Fahrenheit and place a skillet in it.
2. Blend the ginger, garlic, sesame oil, lime juice, lime zest, honey, soy sauce, and cilantro.
3. Once smooth, place in the fridge.
4. Fill a saucepan with 4 quarts of water and place it on the stove.
5. Take out another pan or skillet and place it on the heat.
6. Spray it with oil and add the mushrooms.
7. Cook until browned, then place them to the side.
8. Once the mushrooms are out of the pan, place the salmon in it. If you need to add more oil, do so.
9. Cook for about 6 minutes before turning over and cooking the other side. Cook for the same amount of time.
10. Once it is done, let it cool and then place in the fridge.
11. Once the water has come to a boil, add the snow peas.
12. Only cook them for about 2 minutes. Remove them with tongs or a slotted spoon and rinse them under cold water.
13. Add the noodles to the boiling water and cook for about 10 to 15 minutes.
14. Once the noodles are done, drain them and run them under cold water.
15. Place everything that has finished cooking in the fridge to cool. Leave everything to chill for about an hour before assembling the salad.
16. Once everything has chilled, toss the noodles in the dressing you made in step 2.
17. Add in the mushrooms, snow peas, cilantro, and bok choy. Toss everything together.
18. Add the salmon to the dish by flaking it over the salad.
19. If you are not serving it immediately, place it in the fridge until you are ready to serve.

Seared Salmon and Chickpea Salad

Cal 456 — GLUTEN-FREE

Difficulty: Normal
Preparation time: 15 minutes
Cook time: 15 minutes
Servings: 4

Nutrition per serving (g)

Fat	Saturates	Carbs	Sugars	Protein
17	3	8	8	36

Ingredients

- Spray olive oil
- 16 oz salmon filet
- 2 large carrots, peeled and diced
- 2 ribs celery. diced
- ½ large green bell pepper, diced
- 2 medium yellow squash, seeded and diced
- 2, 15 oz cans no salt added chickpeas, drained and rinsed
- 1 teaspoon paprika
- 1 teaspoon dried rosemary
- 1 teaspoon dried oregano
- ½ teaspoon salt
- 1 tablespoon olive oil
- 1 tablespoon white wine vinegar

Method

1. Preheat the oven to 425 degrees Fahrenheit and place a skillet in it to heat up.
2. Once the skillet is hot, spray it with some oil. Place the salmon skin side down and place it in the oven.
3. Let it cook for about 5 minutes and then turn it.
4. Cook on the other side for the same amount of time.
5. Once it is done, take it out of the oven. Let it cool for a few minutes before placing it in the fridge.
6. Toss the carrots, celery, green pepper, squash, chickpeas, paprika, rosemary, oregano, and salt together. Leave it to stay cold in the fridge.
7. After the salmon has been in the fridge for about 15 minutes, take it out. Peel the skin of the fish.
8. Flake the salmon and fold it into the salad. You can cut up the skin and add it to the salad as well.
9. Pour over the vinegar and olive oil and toss before serving.

Spring Vegetable Quinoa Salad

Cal 181
VEGAN

Difficulty: Normal
Preparation time: 10 minutes
Cook time: 5 minutes
Servings: 2

Nutrition per serving (g)

Fat	Saturates	Carbs	Sugars	Protein
4.5	0.5	28.5	3.5	7.5

Ingredients

- 1 cup asparagus spears, cut into 3-inch pieces
- 1/2 cup peas, fresh or frozen
- 1 cup cooked quinoa
- 2 cups arugula
- 1/2 cup radishes, sliced thinly
- 1/4 cup fresh bazil leaves, roughly chopped
- 1 tablespoon apple cider vinegar
- 1 teaspoon dijon mustard
- 1 tablespoon olive oil

Method

1. Place a pan on the heat and place it in the asparagus and peas. Cover them with water and bring to a boil.
2. Cook for about a minute or until the asparagus turns a bright green color.
3. Remove from the heat, drain, and run under cold water.
4. Pour the asparagus and peas into a bowl, along with the quinoa, arugula, radishes, and bazil. Toss together.
5. Make a dressing with the apple cider vinegar, dijon mustard, and olive oil. Whisk together with a fork.
6. Pour the dressing over the salad and toss.
7. Place in the fridge until you are ready to serve.

Light Avocado Chicken Salad

Cal 174

Difficulty: Easy
Preparation time: 10 minutes
Cook time: 30 minutes
Servings: 4

Nutrition per serving (g)

Fat	Saturates	Carbs	Sugars	Protein
7	1	6	2	23

Ingredients

- 1 large chicken breast, about 2 cups shredded
- Garlic powder, to taste
- 1 small avocado, mashed
- 2 tablespoon plain nonfat Greek yogurt
- 1 teaspoon rice wine vinegar (or to taste)
- ¼ teaspoon garlic powder
- ½ teaspoon onion powder
- ½ cup diced celery, about 1 rib

Method

1. Preheat the oven to 350 degrees Fahrenheit.
2. Place the chicken breast on a baking sheet and sprinkle over the garlic powder.
3. Cover with foil and bake for about 30 minutes.
4. Once the chicken has finished cooking, remove from the oven and let cool.
5. Once cool. Shred with a fork.
6. Peel and mash the avocado.
7. Fold in the yogurt, rice wine vinegar, and garlic powder.
8. Pour in the chicken, along with the onion powder and celery.
9. Mix all of this together and store it in the fridge until you are ready to serve.
10. Serve over a bed of lettuce leaves or even use it as a sandwich filling. It is also delicious just eating it on its own.

Mango Chicken Salad

Cal 238 **GLUTEN-FREE**

Difficulty: Normal
Preparation time: 15 minutes
Cook time: 15 minutes
Servings: 4

Nutrition per serving (g)

Fat	Saturates	Carbs	Sugars	Protein
5	1	20	14	28

Ingredients

- 4 cups water
- 1 lb boneless skinless chicken breasts
- 2 large ribs celery, diced
- 1 large mango, peeled and diced
- ½ red bell pepper, diced
- ¼ cup slivered almonds
- 2 tablespoons fresh dill
- ½ cup reduced-fat mayonnaise
- 2 tablespoons orange juice
- ¼ teaspoon salt

Method

1. Simmer some water over medium heat and poach the chicken in it for about 15 minutes.
2. Pull the chicken out and allow it to rest for about 10 minutes.
3. Once cool, cut into cubes and place in the fridge for 30 minutes.
4. Add the chicken and the rest of the ingredients to a bowl and toss.
5. Serve cold.

Apricot Caprese Salad

Cal 331

GLUTEN-FREE
VEGETARIAN

Difficulty: Easy
Preparation time: 5 minutes
Cook time: 0 minutes
Servings: 4

Nutrition per serving (g)

Fat	Saturates	Carbs	Sugars	Protein
32	7	5.5	4	7.5

Ingredients

- 8 fresh or canned apricot slices
- 8 slices part-skim mozzarella cheese (1oz each)
- 8 fresh basil leaves
- 8 teaspoon extra virgin olive oil
- ¼ teaspoon fresh or dried oregano

Method

1. Layer the apricot and cheese slices.
2. Chop the basil and mix it with the oil. Drizzle it over the apricot and cheese.
3. Sprinkle with oregano.
4. Serve.

Waldorf Salad

Cal 123

GLUTEN-FREE
VEGETARIAN

Difficulty: Normal
Preparation time: 15 minutes
Cook time: 0 minutes
Servings: 8

Nutrition per serving (g)

Fat	Saturates	Carbs	Sugars	Protein
6	1	18	14	1

Ingredients

- 2 medium granny smith apples, cored and cut into ¼ inch cubes
- 1 medium red delicious apple, cored and cut into ¼ inch cubes
- 1 cup celery, cut into large dice
- ¼ cup walnuts, coarsely chopped
- ¼ cup raisins
- ¼ cup low-fat mayonnaise
- ¼ cup low-fat sour cream
- 1 ½ teaspoons honey

Method

1. Add all the ingredients into a bowl and mix.
2. Chill in the fridge for 2 hours before serving.

Tuna Potato Salad

Cal 153 GLUTEN-FREE

Difficulty: Easy
Preparation time: 15 minutes
Cook time: 45 minutes
Servings: 6

Nutrition per serving (g)

Fat	Saturates	Carbs	Sugars	Protein
3	1	21	4	11

Ingredients

- 3 quarts water
- 1 pound Yukon Gold potatoes
- 8 oz carrots peeled and cut into ¼ inch dice
- 2 large hard-boiled eggs, cut into small dice
- 1 cup frozen peas, thawed
- 1, 5 oz no salt added canned tuna in water, drained
- 4 tablespoons reduced-fat mayonnaise
- ¼ teaspoon salt
- 2 teaspoons paprika

Method

1. Place a pot of water on the stove to boil, and then add the carrots.
2. Allow the carrots to cook for 15 minutes.
3. Remove and add the potatoes and cook for 30 minutes.
4. Drain, and allow the potatoes to cool. Peel the skin and then cut into cubes.
5. Place all the ingredients in a bowl and mix together.
6. Chill then serve.

Main Meals

Cashew Chicken	GLUTEN-FREE	98
Chicken with Sauteed Mushrooms		100
Mango Tilapia	GLUTEN-FREE	101
Lentil burgers	VEGETARIAN	102
Black Bean Burgers	VEGETARIAN	103
Chicken and Red Potatoes		104
Crispy Peanut Shrimp		105
Steak and Blackberry Glaze	GLUTEN-FREE	106
Kung Pao Chicken	GLUTEN-FREE	108
Crispy Peanut Shrimp		110
Pork Chops and Apples	GLUTEN-FREE	111
Carbonara		112
Papaya Whitefish with Ginger		113
Tomato Sauce-Free Lasagna		114
Turkey Meatballs		116
Quinoa Stuffed Chicken Roll-Ups	GLUTEN-FREE	117
Glazed Salmon and Lentils	GLUTEN-FREE	118
Pecan Crusted Trout	GLUTEN-FREE	119

Mac and Cheese with Salmon	120
Chicken Parmesan	121
Juicy Turkey and Mushroom Burgers	122
Buttermilk Chicken	123
Chicken Tetrazzini	124
Cauliflower Steak	126
Shrimp and Pea Stir Fry	127
Creamy Mac and Cheese — VEGETARIAN	128
Fettuccine Alfredo — VEGETARIAN	129
Gnocchi — VEGETARIAN	130

This section is labeled as "Main Meals" because they can be used as either dinner or lunch recipes. You can make extra for dinner and take the leftovers for lunch. Some of these are so delicious that there won't even be any leftovers for lunch.

Dinner is a great time to try new recipes because you have a bit more time, especially over the weekend. There are recipes for all types and all situations. Whether you are making food for just you or hosting your friends, you will find something you love. I would challenge you to try something that you never have before. You never know what might turn into your new favorite weeknight meal.

Cashew Chicken

Cal 500 GLUTEN-FREE

Difficulty: Normal
Preparation time: 15 minutes
Cook time: 45 minutes
Servings: 2

Nutrition per serving (g)

Fat	Saturates	Carbs	Sugars	Protein
18	3.5	51	6	33

Ingredients

- 1 cup frozen shelled edamame, soybeans
- 2 cups water
- 1 cup brown rice, uncooked
- 2 teaspoons dark sesame oil
- 1 teaspoon of onion powder or to taste
- ¼ teaspoon of garlic powder
- 1 lb boneless skinless chicken thighs cut into ½ inch cubes
- ½ cup raw cashews
- 1 tablespoon fresh ginger, peeled and minced
- ½ cup no salt added vegetable broth
- 2 tablespoon gluten-free tamari sauce
- 1 tablespoon maple syrup

Method

1. Rinse the edamame beans in cool water and set aside.
2. Boil some water in a medium saucepan and add the rice.
3. Reduce the heat so that it simmers and let it cook for about 40 minutes.
4. Make sure that all the water does not boil away. Once there is a little bit of water left in the saucepan, take it off the heat and let it stand.
5. While you wait for the rice to cook, place some oil in a skillet and set it on medium heat.
6. Add the garlic and cook until it has softened, then add the onion powder.
7. Add in the chicken thighs and cashew nuts.
8. Once the outside of the chicken has browned, add in the broth, tamari sauce, and maple syrup.
9. Let it cook for a further 2 minutes and then add the edamame beans.
10. Let this all cook together until the chicken has fully cooked through. This should take about 10 minutes.
11. Serve the chicken over the rice.

Chicken with Sauteed Mushrooms

Cal 293

Difficulty: Normal
Preparation time: 10 minutes
Cook time: 20 to 25 minutes
Servings: 4

Nutrition per serving (g)

Fat	Saturates	Carbs	Sugars	Protein
18.2	6.8	8.5	0.8	25.5

Ingredients

- 1 pound boneless, skinless chicken breasts
- ⅓ cup whole wheat flour
- 2 tablespoons olive oil
- 3 tablespoons butter
- 2 cups mushrooms, sliced
- ⅓ cup white wine or chicken broth
- Salt

Method

1. Slice the chicken breasts in half, lengthways. You should have thin pieces of chicken.
2. Season the chicken.
3. Place the flour in a bowl and dip each piece of chicken in it.
4. Heat some oil in a pan and add the chicken. Let the chicken brown for about 3 minutes on each side.
5. Once the chicken is done, remove it from the pan and put it to one side.
6. Turn the heat down and toss in the butter and mushrooms.
7. Saute the mushrooms until they are soft. This should take about 5 minutes.
8. Add the wine or broth into the pan and stir.
9. Place the chicken back into the pan. The sauce should thicken. It should only take a few minutes.
10. Once the sauce has thickened, you can serve.

Mango Tilapia

Cal 406

GLUTEN-FREE

Difficulty: Easy
Preparation time: 10 minutes
Cook time: 15 minutes
Servings: 4

Nutrition per serving (g)

Fat	Saturates	Carbs	Sugars	Protein
13.5	2.5	34	10.5	38

Ingredients

- 1 cup of long grain rice
- 2 tablespoons of mango juice
- 1 tablespoon of grated ginger
- 2 teaspoons of honey
- 3 tablespoons olives oil
- 1 pound of mango chunks, fresh or canned
- 1 small English cucumber, chopped
- ¼ cup of chopped red sweet pepper*
- 4, 6-oz tilapia filets

Method

1. Put a pot of salted water on to boil and cook the rice according to the package instructions.
2. Mix manjo juice, ginger, honey, 2 tablespoons of olive oil, and salt in a bowl.
3. Pour the liquid over the manjo chunks, English cucumber, and sweet pepper. Toss this thoroughly.
4. Place a skillet on the stove to heat up. Add in the remaining oil.
5. Season the tilapia fillets with salt. Place them in the pan and cook for about 2 or 3 minutes on each side.
6. Serve the tilapia with a side of rice and relish.

The sweet red pepper should not trigger any acid reflux. However, if you are worried or have reacted to it, then it is better to leave it out.

Lentil burgers

Cal 252 VEGETARIAN

Difficulty: Easy
Preparation time: 10 minutes
Cook time: 10 minutes
Servings: 4

Nutrition per serving (g)

Fat	Saturates	Carbs	Sugars	Protein
7	1.5	20	3	17

Ingredients

- 2 cups cooked lentils
- ½ cup dried bread crumbs
- 2 egg whites
- ¼ cup grated carrot
- ¾ cup chopped kale
- 1 or 2 tablespoons chopped dried onion (according to preference)
- ¼ teaspoon kosher salt
- ½ teaspoon cumin
- ⅓ cup grated sharp cheddar cheese
- Iceberg lettuce
- Honey mustard dressing
- Whole wheat hamburger buns (toasted)
- 1 tablespoon Canola or olive oil

Method

1. Mash all the ingredients, except the oil, together in a bowl.
2. Form the patties using your hands. Chill for an hour
3. Heat the oil in a pan and cook the patties for 3 minutes on each side or until golden brown.
4. Serve on a whole wheat bun or a bed of lettuce.

Black Bean Burgers

Cal 344 VEGETARIAN	**Difficulty:** Easy **Preparation time:** 10 minutes **Cook time:** 15 minutes **Servings:** 6			

Nutrition per serving (g)

Fat	Saturates	Carbs	Sugars	Protein
13	1.2	46.5	3	16

Ingredients

- 2, 15 oz cans of black beans drained
- 2 eggs
- ⅓ cup of green pepper, chopped
- 2 tablespoons of flour
- 2 tablespoons of minced cilantro
- 1 teaspoon of ground cumin
- ½ teaspoon of ground coriander
- ¼ teaspoon of salt
- ½ cup of baked tortilla chips, crushed
- ¼ cup of vegetable oil
- Iceberg lettuce
- 6 whole wheat buns

Method

1. Drain the black beans and place them on paper towels to dry out for about 20 minutes.
2. Once they have dried, mash the beans up with the eggs, tortilla chips, and seasoning.
3. Shape the mixture into patties and place them in the fridge for about an hour.
4. Once the patties have firmed up a bit, place a pan on the stove to heat up.
5. Pour in the oil and fry the patties for about 4 to 5 minutes on each side. They should be nice and crisp.
6. Place the patties on paper towels to drain any excess oil.
7. Build the burger with the bun, a patty, and lettuce. You can add the condiments you choose.

Chicken and Red Potatoes

Cal 412

Difficulty: Normal
Preparation time: 15 minutes
Cook time: 40 minutes
Servings: 4

Nutrition per serving (g)

Fat	Saturates	Carbs	Sugars	Protein
22	7	19	3	34

Ingredients

- 2 cups red potatoes cut into one inch cubes
- 2 large carrots, peeled and sliced into 1 inch pieces
- 1 tablespoon low fat butter, melted
- ¼ teaspoon kosher salt
- ¼ teaspoon turmeric
- 2 cups grilled chicken meat shredded
- ½ teaspoon dried rosemary
- ⅓ cup pitted green olives (optional)
- 2 tablespoons apple cider vinegar
- 2 tablespoons fresh parsley

Method

1. Switch the oven on and let it heat up to 425 degrees Fahrenheit.
2. Place the potatoes and carrots into a bowl and toss them with the melted butter, turmeric, and salt.
3. Pour them out onto a baking sheet. Spread the vegetables out so that they are as flat as possible in the tray.
4. Place them in the pre-heated oven and let them bake for 35 minutes or until the vegetables are all soft and cooked through.
5. Stir the vegetables once halfway through cooking.
6. Once they are done, pour them into a casserole dish.
7. Add the chicken, olives, rosemary, and apple cider vinegar. Mix through well.
8. Place the casserole dish into the oven and bake for 15 minutes.
9. Remove from the oven and garnish with the fresh parsley. Serve hot.

Steak and Blackberry Glaze

Cal 384
GLUTEN-FREE

Difficulty: Normal
Preparation time: 15 minutes
Cook time: 35 minutes
Servings: 2

Nutrition per serving (g)

Fat	Saturates	Carbs	Sugars	Protein
13	6	30	20	30

Ingredients

- 2 tablespoons blackberry preserves
- 1 tablespoon light brown sugar
- 4 tablespoons white wine
- ¼ teaspoon salt
- ⅛ teaspoon dried marjoram leaves
- Spray olive oil
- 1 lb crimini or wild mushrooms, cut in quarters
- 1 teaspoon olive oil
- 8 oz flank steak
- 2 teaspoons unsalted butter

Method

1. Switch on the oven and let it heat up at 375 degrees Fahrenheit.
2. Mix the preserve, sugar, wine, marjoram, and salt in a bowl.
3. Spray a pan with olive oil spray and place it on the stove to heat up.
4. Place the mushrooms in the pan and let it cook for about 20 minutes. Stir occasionally so that it doesn't stick to the pan.
5. Remove the mushrooms from the pan and set them aside.
6. Add some olive oil to the pan and increase the heat to high.
7. Place the steak in the pan. You should hear a sizzle.
8. Spoon about half of the blackberry sauce you made earlier on top of the steak.
9. Let the steak cook for about 6 minutes before turning.
10. Pour the remaining sauce over the other side of the steak.

11. Let the steak cook for another 5 to 7 minutes before removing from the pan and setting it aside to rest.

12. While the steak is resting, place the pan back on the heat and add the mushrooms.

13. Add the butter and wine and mix together. Once the butter has melted, lower the heat.

14. Once everything has combined, remove the pan from the heat.

15. Slice the steak and pour the sauce and mushrooms over it to serve.

Kung Pao Chicken

Cal 452 GLUTEN-FREE

Difficulty: Normal
Preparation time: 10 minutes
Cook time: 40 minutes
Servings: 4

Nutrition per serving (g)

Fat	Saturates	Carbs	Sugars	Protein
16	4	43	31	26

Ingredients

- 16 oz chicken breast, cut into 1-inch cubes
- 2 teaspoons low-sodium soy sauce or gluten-free tamari sauce
- 2 teaspoons sake or sweet white wine
- 1 teaspoon sesame oil
- 2 teaspoons rice vinegar
- 2 teaspoons honey
- 1 teaspoon cornstarch
- 2 cups water
- 1 cup jasmine rice
- 1 tablespoon sesame oil
- 1-inch piece of ginger root, minced
- 2 tablespoons rice vinegar
- 2 tablespoons low-sodium soy sauce or gluten-free tamari sauce
- ¾ cup water
- ¼ cup dry roasted peanuts, chopped coarsely

Method

1. Mix 2 teaspoons low-sodium soy sauce, sake, 1 teaspoon sesame oil, rice vinegar, honey, and cornstarch in a bowl.

2. Add the chicken to the marinade and put it in the fridge for the time being.

3. While you are waiting for the beef to marinade, cook the rice according to the instructions on the package.

4. Don't stir the rice or let all the water boil away.

5. When there is a minimal amount of water left in the rice, take it off the stove.

6. Cover the pot and let it stand for 5 minutes.

7. Heat the sesame oil in a pan and add the ginger.

8. Let the ginger cook for about a minute before adding the chicken.

9. Cook the chicken until it has browned. Add the rice vinegar and soy or tamari sauce.

10. Toss the chicken frequently until it has almost finished cooking, then add the water to loosen the sauce.

11. Let cook for another minute or so.

12. Plate up the rice and serve the chicken over it. Sprinkle peanuts over the dish.

Crispy Peanut Shrimp

Cal 394

Difficulty: Easy
Preparation time: 10 minutes
Cook time: 20 minutes
Servings: 4

Nutrition per serving (g)

Fat	Saturates	Carbs	Sugars	Protein
18	2	28	3	30

Ingredients

- 1 tablespoon peanut butter
- 2 tablespoons light coconut milk
- 1 tablespoon tamari sauce
- 1 teaspoon cream of tartar mixed with 2 tablespoons of water
- 1 ¼ cups panko crumbs
- 16 oz large shrimp, peeled and deveined
- 3 tablespoons sesame oil

Method

1. Take out a bowl and mix in the peanut butter, tamari sauce, cream of tartar mixture, and coconut milk.
2. Pour the panko crumbs into a flat plate.
3. Take each one of your shrimp, dip them into the sauce, and then into the crumbs.
4. Coat the shrimp on both sides and lightly pat watch one so that the panko crumbs stick to them.
5. Pour the oil into a pan and set it to medium heat.
6. Once the oil is nice and hot, drop the shrimp in. Make sure you hear a sizzle. If not, the pan is not hot enough. Test one shrimp before pouring all into the pan.
7. Cook the shrimp for about 8 minutes on each side.
8. Once the shrimp are cooked through, you can remove them from the pan.
9. Enjoy on their own or on the top of a salad.

Pork Chops and Apples

Cal 318
GLUTEN-FREE

Difficulty: Normal
Preparation time: 15 minutes
Cook time: 35 minutes
Servings: 2

Nutrition per serving (g)

Fat	Saturates	Carbs	Sugars	Protein
9	3.5	31	25	25

Ingredients

- 1 teaspoon unsalted butter
- 2 medium granny smith apples, peeled and sliced
- 2 teaspoons sugar
- ¼ teaspoon salt
- 1 teaspoon maple syrup
- 1 tablespoon apple cider vinegar
- ¼ cup sweet, white wine
- ¼ teaspoon dried thyme
- ¼ cup water
- 2, 4 oz center cut pork chops, trimmed of all fat
- 1 teaspoon oil or spray oil

Method

1. Place a pan on the stove and put the butter in.
2. Once the butter has melted, add the apples and the sugar.
3. Let the apples caramelize. It should take about 20 minutes. Turn occasionally.
4. As the apples start to soften up, add the salt, maple syrup, apple cider vinegar, wine, and thyme. Let everything cook together.
5. Reduce the heat and let the apples simmer for about 10 minutes.
6. While you are waiting for your apples, heat up the oven to 400 degrees Fahrenheit.
7. Place a skillet in the oven to heat up.
8. Once the skillet is hot (about 10 minutes), season the pork chops and place them in the hot skillet with the oil.
9. Place the chops in the oven for about 8 minutes. Turn and then cook on the other side for a further 10 minutes.
10. Once everything is done, serve the chops topped with the caramelized apples. You can also serve with a side salad or mashed potatoes.

Carbonara

Cal 482

Difficulty: Normal
Preparation time: 10 minutes
Cook time: 20 minutes
Servings: 2

Nutrition per serving (g)

Fat	Saturates	Carbs	Sugars	Protein
17	6	54	4	28

Ingredients

- 3 quarts water
- 4 oz whole wheat or gluten-free linguine
- 2 teaspoons olive oil
- ¼ teaspoons of garlic powder
- 2 oz prosciutto, diced
- 1 cup frozen peas, thawed
- ¼ cup white wine
- 2 large eggs
- 1 oz parmesan cheese, grated

Method

1. Place a large pot of water on the stove to boil.
2. When the water is boiling, add the pasta and salt. Cook for as long as the packet instructs.
3. While the pasta is cooking, put a pan on the heat.
4. Add the oil, garlic, and prosciutto. Let it cook until the prosciutto is crispy.
5. Then add the peas and let it cook for a few minutes.
6. While that is cooking, get a bowl out.
7. Whisk the eggs and parmesan together.
8. Once the pasta is cooked, add the white wine to the pan and then add the pasta. Use tongs so that some of the pasta water transfers with it.
9. Increase the heat to about a medium temperature.
10. Pour the egg mixture into the pan and mix briskly with a plastic spatula.
11. Add a few more spoons of the pasta water and keep mixing until the egg turns into a creamy sauce. You will have to do this fast so the eggs don't scramble.
12. Dish up and serve.

Papaya Whitefish with Ginger

Cal 182

Difficulty: Normal
Preparation time: 10 minutes
Cook time: 20 minutes
Servings: 2

Nutrition per serving (g)

Fat	Saturates	Carbs	Sugars	Protein
3	1	6	4	30

Ingredients

- 1 teaspoon sesame oil
- ½ teaspoon ground ginger
- ¼ cup papaya juice
- ¼ teaspoon salt
- Spray olive oil
- 2, 6 oz whitefish filets
- 1 teaspoon cornstarch
- 4 tablespoons water
- 2 tablespoons fresh cilantro leaves

Method

1. Take out a bowl and add the sesame oil, papaya juice, ginger, and salt.
2. Place a pan on the stove, add some oil to the pan, and let it heat up.
3. Once the pan is hot, add the fish. Cook for 4 minutes on each side.
4. While the fish is cooking, take out a bowl for the cornstarch and 4 tablespoons of water.
5. Mix up the ingredients until it forms a paste. Then add the papaya sauce.
6. Add the mixture to the fish and coat both sides. Let it cook for a few more minutes to let the flavor seep in.
7. Plate up the fish and pour the sauce over and serve.

Tomato Sauce-Free Lasagna

Cal 314

Difficulty: Normal
Preparation time: 25 minutes
Cook time: 35 minutes
Servings: 10

Nutrition per serving (g)

Fat	Saturates	Carbs	Sugars	Protein
3	1	6	4	30

Ingredients

- 12 oz wide lasagna noodles
- 12 oz very lean ground beef (ground round or ground sirloin)
- Nonstick cooking spray
- 1/2 cup low-sodium beef broth
- 1/4 cup low-fat cream cheese
- 1 1/4 cups skim milk or 1% milk, divided
- 1 tablespoon all-purpose flour
- 2 tablespoons butter or margarine
- 1/2 cup shredded good-quality Parmesan cheese
- Salt
- 1 1/2 cups grated skim mozzarella cheese

Method

1. Preheat an oven to 375 degrees Fahrenheit.
2. Place a large pot of water on the stove to boil. Add the lasagne sheets and cook until just tender.
3. Place a pan on the stove and spray with cooking spray. Once hot, add the beef. Cook until browned.
4. Add the beef broth to the pan and cook it together until the broth reduces a bit.
5. Combine the cream cheese, ¼ cup milk, and flour in a bowl.
6. Slowly pour in the remaining milk and beat until combined.
7. Place the butter in a saucepan and set it on the heat. Once the butter has melted, add the cream cheese mixture you just made.
8. Let the sauce heat through and thicken for about 5 minutes. Stir continuously.
9. Add in the parmesan cheese and season with salt. Stir until the cheese has melted. Remove from the heat.
10. Once the lasagne sheets are done cooking, drain them and set them aside.
11. Get out an ovenproof dish to assemble your lasagne in.

12. Spread 1 cup of the white sauce on the bottom of the dish and place 3 lasagne sheets on top to cover it.

13. Spoon over half of the beef, followed by more white sauce and then another 3 pasta sheets.

14. Keep doing this until you have run out of pasta sheets. The last layer should be a layer of white sauce.

15. Sprinkle some mozzarella cheese over the top and bake for about 25 minutes or until the top is bubbly and the cheese has turned golden.

16. Cut up into equal portions and serve.

Turkey Meatballs

Cal 285

Difficulty: Normal
Preparation time: 10 minutes
Cook time: 25 minutes
Servings: 4

Nutrition per serving (g)

Fat	Saturates	Carbs	Sugars	Protein
7.5	2.5	13	3	36

Ingredients

- 1 pound ground turkey meat
- 1 package (10 oz) frozen spinach
- 1 egg, beaten
- 1 tablespoon low-fat milk
- 1 cup soft bread crumbs
- ½ teaspoon turmeric
- ½ teaspoon ginger
- 1 tablespoon onion powder

Method

1. Preheat the oven to 400 degrees Fahrenheit.
2. Squeeze the spinach dry.
3. Mix the spinach, egg, milk, bread crumbs, seasonings, and onion powder.
4. Add the turkey meat, mix and shape the meatballs.
5. Place on a greased baking sheet and bake in the oven for 25 minutes.
6. Serve.

Quinoa Stuffed Chicken Roll-Ups

Cal 112
GLUTEN-FREE

Difficulty: Normal
Preparation time: 15 minutes
Cook time: 40 minutes
Servings: 4

Nutrition per serving (g)

Fat	Saturates	Carbs	Sugars	Protein
3	1	5	1	25

Ingredients

- 2 tablespoons quinoa, dry
- ½ medium carrot, julienned
- ¼ cup broccoli stalks, julienned
- 2 medium boneless, skinless chicken breasts
- ¼ teaspoon salt
- ¼ teaspoon oregano, dry
- ½ cup spinach, chopped
- 2 tablespoons feta cheese, crumbled

Method

1. Preheat the oven to 350 degrees Fahrenheit.
2. Place a pot on the stove and cook the quinoa according to the instructions on the package.
3. Use a steamer basket or colander placed inside a pot of water to steam the carrots and broccoli.
4. Pound the chicken breast until it is about ¼ of an inch in thickness.
5. Spray a baking sheet with cooking spray and lay the chicken breasts on it.
6. Rub the chicken with salt on both sides.
7. Once the vegetables and quinoa are all cooked, layer them on top of the chicken breast.
8. Layer the spinach, and feta cheese.
9. Make sure that everything is in the middle and is not falling to the sides.
10. Roll one side of the chicken breast over and then the other. Secure it with toothpicks or tie it with some twine.
11. Place a pan on the heat, and once hot, brown the chicken in it. It should only take about 5 minutes.
12. Transfer the chicken back onto the baking tray and let it roast in the oven for 15 minutes.
13. Once the chicken is ready, take it out of the oven and let it cool slightly before slicing and serving.

Glazed Salmon and Lentils

Cal 512 — GLUTEN-FREE

Difficulty: Normal
Preparation time: 10 minutes
Cook time: 30 minutes
Servings: 2

Nutrition per serving (g)

Fat	Saturates	Carbs	Sugars	Protein
18	3	50	16	38

Ingredients

- Spray olive oil
- 1 large celery, diced
- 2 medium carrots, peeled and diced
- ½ cup red lentils
- 1 cup water
- ½ cup low sodium chicken or vegetable broth
- ¼ teaspoon salt
- 1 teaspoon dried marjoram or oregano
- 1 tablespoon extra virgin olive oil
- 2, 4 oz salmon filets
- 2 tablespoons maple syrup

Method

1. Place a skillet on the heat and heat up the oil.
2. Once hot, add the celery and carrots. Let this cook for about 5 minutes, making sure to stir every so often.
3. Then pour in the lentils, water, chicken stock, salt, and marjoram or oregano. Stir and let it simmer.
4. Cook until the lentils have softened, which should take about 20 minutes.
5. While the lentils are cooking away, preheat the oven to 375 degrees Fahrenheit.
6. Spray a pan or skillet with nonstick spray or add a bit of oil to it. Place it in the oven to heat up.
7. Once the pan is hot, place the salmon in it and top with maple syrup. Place it back in the oven for about 4 minutes.
8. Take the salmon out, turn it, and top the other side with maple syrup. Place it back in the oven to cook for a further 5 minutes.
9. The lentils should be done at this point. If there is any leftover liquid, drain the lentils.
10. Serve by laying the salmon over a bed of lentils. Any liquid that is left over in the salmon pan can be poured over the dish as a sauce.

Pecan Crusted Trout

Cal 445 — GLUTEN-FREE

Difficulty: Normal
Preparation time: 10 minutes
Cook time: 15 minutes
Servings: 2

Nutrition per serving (g)

Fat	Saturates	Carbs	Sugars	Protein
13	4	11	7	26

Ingredients

- 1 ½ oz raw pecans
- 1 tablespoon fresh sage
- 1 ½ teaspoons fresh rosemary
- ⅛ teaspoon salt
- ¼ teaspoon smoked paprika
- 1 tablespoon maple syrup
- 2, 4 oz boneless trout filets, leave the skin on
- 1 tablespoon olive oil
- ¼ cup white wine
- 1 teaspoon unsalted butter

Method

1. Preheat the oven to 375 degrees Fahrenheit and place a skillet in the oven to heat up.
2. Blend up the pecans, sage, rosemary, salt, and paprika, in a food processor or mini-chopper.
3. Pulse until you have a sand-like consistency.
4. Pour out the mixture into a bowl and add the syrup. Mix well.
5. Take the skillet out of the oven and pour in the oil. Place it back in the oven for about a minute.
6. Take the fish and pat the pecan mixture onto the skin. Make sure it sticks well.
7. Take the skillet out of the oven and palace the trout in it, skin side down.
8. Place it back in the oven and let it cook for about 5 minutes.
9. Set the oven to broil and let it cook for a further 3 to 5 minutes.
10. Once cooked, place the fish on plates and set aside.
11. Take the same skillet and place it on medium heat.
12. Pour in the white wine and stir gently for a few seconds.
13. Add in the butter. Once it is melted, pour the sauce over the trout and serve.

Mac and Cheese with Salmon

Cal 463

Difficulty: Easy
Preparation time: 5 minutes
Cook time: 45 minutes
Servings: 4

Nutrition per serving (g)

Fat	Saturates	Carbs	Sugars	Protein
15	7	49	3	35

Ingredients

- 4 quarts water
- 8 oz whole wheat penne pasta or shells
- 2 large eggs
- ½ cup 2% milk
- ¼ teaspoon dried tarragon
- 4 oz reduced-fat Monterey Jack cheese, grated
- 8 oz salmon, skinless; sliced into thin strips
- 1 cup frozen peas
- ¼ teaspoon salt

Method

1. Set the oven to 375 degrees Fahrenheit to heat up.
2. Place a large pot of water on the stove to boil. Place pasta in and cook according to the instructions on the package.
3. Once the pasta is slightly underdone, take it off the heat and drain it.
4. Whisk together the eggs and milk.
5. Once combined, add in the tarragon, cheese, salmon, peas, and salt. Gently fold.
6. Pour the mixture over the pasta and make sure it is all mixed through.
7. Pour it into an oven-safe dish and bake for about 30 minutes.
8. Remove from the oven and let cook for a few minutes before serving.

Chicken Parmesan

Cal 380

Difficulty: Normal
Preparation time: 10 minutes
Cook time: 30 minutes
Servings: 2

Nutrition per serving (g)

Fat	Saturates	Carbs	Sugars	Protein
17	9	15	3	42

Ingredients

- 1 slice whole wheat bread
- ½ teaspoon dried oregano
- ½ teaspoon dried basil
- ⅛ teaspoon dried tarragon
- ¼ teaspoon dried marjoram
- 1 large egg
- 2 tablespoons all-purpose flour or garbanzo flour
- 2 teaspoons unsalted butter
- 2, 4 oz boneless, skinless chicken breasts
- 1 oz Parmigiano Reggiano, grated
- 6 tablespoons low-acid tomato sauce
- 2 oz low-moisture mozzarella, shredded

Method

1. Set the oven to 300 degrees Fahrenheit and place the bread in there until it dries out and gets crispy.
2. Take the bread out and let it cool for a few minutes.
3. Increase the heat of the oven to 375 degrees Fahrenheit and place a skillet in it.
4. Pulse the bread, oregano, basil, tarragon, and marjoram until you have a crumb.
5. Take out a bowl and whisk up an egg.
6. Place some flour into a plate and dip the chicken breast into it.
7. Take the breasts and dip them into the egg, and then into the breadcrumbs.
8. Take the skillet from the oven and add some butter to it. Place the chicken breasts in the skillet and put it back in the oven.
9. Leave it to cook for about 12 minutes.
10. Turn them over and sprinkle over some grated parmesan. Place it back in the oven for another 2 or 3 minutes.
11. Place 3 tablespoons of tomato sauce per breast.
12. Sprinkle over the mozzarella and place it back in the oven until the cheese has melted.
13. Serve hot.

Juicy Turkey and Mushroom Burgers

Cal 85

Difficulty: Normal
Preparation time: 15 minutes
Cook time: 10 minutes
Servings: 6

Nutrition per serving (g)

Fat	Saturates	Carbs	Sugars	Protein
3	1	1	1	13

Ingredients

- ¾ pound turkey breast, ground
- ½ cup Baby Bella mushrooms, finely chopped
- 1 tablespoon olive oil
- 1 tablespoon Worcestershire sauce

Method

1. Place the turkey breast, mushrooms, olive oil, and Worcestershire sauce into a bowl. Mix all these ingredients thoroughly.
2. Divide the mixture into 6 equal portions.
3. Roll and flatten into patty shapes. They should be about ½ and inch thick.
4. Place a pan on the stove to heat up. Grease the pan with cooking spray or a small amount of oil.
5. Cook them on medium heat for 5 minutes on each side.
6. Remove from the heat.
7. You can serve on a burger bun or on a bed of lettuce.

Buttermilk Chicken

Cal **409**

Difficulty: Normal
Preparation time: 10 minutes
Cook time: 25 minutes
Servings: 4

Nutrition per serving (g)

Fat	Saturates	Carbs	Sugars	Protein
31	7	8	1	24

Ingredients

- ½ cup all-purpose flour
- 1 teaspoon dried rosemary
- ½ teaspoon dried oregano
- ½ teaspoon dried thyme
- ½ cup nonfat buttermilk
- ⅛ teaspoon hot sauce
- ¼ teaspoon salt
- ½ cup canola oil
- 4 bone-in, skin-on chicken thighs

Method

1. Get out a flat plate and mix the flour, rosemary, oregano, and thyme.
2. In a bowl, mix together the buttermilk, hot sauce, and salt.
3. Place a pan on the stove to heat up with the oil.
4. Dip the chicken into the flour, then the buttermilk mixture, and then back into the flour.
5. Once the oil is hot enough, drop the chicken into the pan.
6. Cook for about 7 minutes and then flip.
7. Let the other side cook for about the same amount of time.
8. Repeat this for all the chicken thighs.
9. Remove the chicken from the oil, once it is cooked. Place it on a plate with paper towels to drain any excess oil.
10. Serve immediately.

Chicken Tetrazzini

Cal 570

Difficulty: Normal
Preparation time: 15 minutes
Cook time: 65 minutes
Servings: 4

Nutrition per serving (g)

Fat	Saturates	Carbs	Sugars	Protein
3	1	1	1	13

Ingredients

- 4 teaspoons olive oil, divided
- 1 lb. cremini mushrooms, quartered
- 4 quarts water
- 8 oz whole wheat linguine
- ¼ cup all-purpose flour
- 1 ½ cups 2% milk
- ½ cup white wine
- 1 cup low sodium chicken stock
- ½ teaspoon dried thyme
- ¼ teaspoon salt
- 2 cups frozen peas
- 12 oz boneless, skinless chicken thighs, diced
- 2 oz Parmigiano Reggiano, grated

Method

1. Put the oven on to 325 degrees Fahrenheit and place a skillet in it to heat up.

2. Once the skillet is nice and hot, add some oil and the mushrooms. Place it back in the oven.

3. Let the mushrooms cook for about 25 minutes. Toss a few times during cooking.

4. Place a pot of water on the stove and let it boil. Add the pasta and cook for about 15 minutes. The pasta should be al dente.

5. Take out another skillet and set it on the heat. Add 3 teaspoons of oil.

6. Once hot add in the flour and mix it all together. It should have a thick consistency.

7. Add the milk about a ½ cup at a time and stir continuously. The sauce will begin to thicken.

8. Pour in the wine, chicken stock, thyme, and salt.

9. Cook for about 2 or 3 minutes and then add the peas and chicken.

10. Keep stirring.

11. Throw in the cooked mushrooms.

12. When the pasta is done cooking, drain it and add it to the sauce.

13. Mix well and pour it into an oven-safe dish.

14. Bake for 40 minutes.

15. Sprinkle the top with parmesan cheese and place it back in the oven until the cheese melts and goes a golden brown color.

Cauliflower Steak

Cal 168

Difficulty: Easy
Preparation time: 5 minutes
Cook time: 50 minutes
Servings: 2

Nutrition per serving (g)

Fat	Saturates	Carbs	Sugars	Protein
13	0	11	4	4

Ingredients

- 1 large head cauliflower
- 3 teaspoon olive oil
- 3 teaspoon unsalted butter
- ⅛ teaspoon salt

Method

1. Preheat the oven to 350 degrees Fahrenheit and palace a skillet in it.
2. Take the cauliflower head and place it on a chopping board, stem side down.
3. Slice it in half, straight down the middle.
4. Cut a 2-inch slice off each of the sides.
5. Reserve the rest of the cauliflower to use in another dish.
6. Remove the stem. The easiest way to do this is to cut a V shape at the base of the cauliflower.
7. Take the skillet out of the oven and add in the olive oil.
8. Place the cauliflower steaks in the pan and palace it in the oven for about 30 minutes. Turn the steaks every 7 minutes, so that both sides are cooked evenly.
9. Remove from the oven and add butter to the skillet.
10. Roast for another 20 minutes. Turning the steaks every few minutes so that both sides brown evenly.
11. Remove from the oven and serve. You can serve this with the sauce of your choosing and a few more veggies if you would like.

Shrimp and Pea Stir Fry

Cal 185

Difficulty: Easy
Preparation time: 10 minutes
Cook time: 10 minutes
Servings: 4

Nutrition per serving (g)

Fat	Saturates	Carbs	Sugars	Protein
8.5	3	7	4	17

Ingredients

- 1 fresh sweet bell pepper (chopped)
- 2 tablespoons finely grated ginger
- ⅔ pound white cabbage (sliced into thin strips)
- 1 tablespoon olive or canola oil
- 1 teaspoon sesame oil
- 1-½ cups frozen peas
- ¾ pound cooked and peeled large shrimp
- 4 tablespoons chopped fresh cilantro

Method

1. Heat up the oils in a pan and add the ginger, bell pepper, and peas.
2. Stir-fry for about 2 minutes then add the cabbage. Cook for another few minutes.
3. Add the shrimp and cook for 2 minutes or until the shrimp are cooked through.
4. take off the heat and stir in cilantro. Serve.

Creamy Mac and Cheese

Cal 308
VEGETARIAN

Difficulty: Easy
Preparation time: 5 minutes
Cook time: 25 minutes
Servings: 4

Nutrition per serving (g)

Fat	Saturates	Carbs	Sugars	Protein
6	3	45	2	21

Ingredients

- 4 quarts water
- 8 oz whole wheat penne pasta
- 2 large eggs
- ½ cup 2% milk
- 5 oz reduced-fat cheddar cheese
- ⅛ teaspoon salt

Method

1. Boil the water in a large pot and cook the pasta according to the package instructions.
2. While the pasta is cooking, start making the sauce.
3. Whisk the milk and eggs in a saucepan.
4. Add the cheese and salt. Stir it all together.
5. Once the pasta is done cooking, add it to the sauce mixture and place the saucepan over medium heat.
6. Stir continuously and don't let the mixture come to a boil.
7. Once the sauce is nice and thick, remove from the heat and serve.

Fettuccine Alfredo

Cal 389 VEGETARIAN

Difficulty: Easy
Preparation time: 5 minutes
Cook time: 25 minutes
Servings: 2

Nutrition per serving (g)

Fat	Saturates	Carbs	Sugars	Protein
12	6	53	5	20

Ingredients

- 1 teaspoon extra virgin olive oil
- ¼ teaspoon garlic powder
- 2 teaspoons all-purpose white flour
- ¾ cup 2% milk
- 1 oz semi-soft goat cheese
- 1 oz Parmigiano-Reggiano, grated
- 4 quarts water
- 4 oz whole wheat fettuccine
- 1 tablespoon parsley, minced

Method

1. Place a pot of water on to boil and cook the pasta according to the directions on the package.
2. Take out a pan and put it over medium heat. Pour the oil in it.
3. Add the garlic powder and stir.
4. Slowly add the flour and cook it for about a minute.
5. Make sure it doesn't burn or brown. It should have a thick consistency.
6. Slowly add the milk and continue stirring.
7. Once all the milk is added and the sauce has begun thickening, add the goat cheese.
8. Once the sauce has a smooth consistency, add the parmesan.
9. Reduce the heat and mix it all together until all the cheese melts. Remove from the heat.
10. Once the pasta has cooked, drain, and add it to the sauce.
11. Coat the pasta thoroughly in the sauce and add some minced parsley to the dish.
12. Serve hot.

Gnocchi

Cal **239** VEGETARIAN	**Difficulty:** Normal **Preparation time:** 20 minutes **Cook time:** 40 minutes **Servings:** 2

Nutrition per serving (g)

Fat	Saturates	Carbs	Sugars	Protein
3	1	45	1	8

Ingredients

- 10 oz Yukon Gold potatoes
- 6 tablespoons all-purpose white flour
- 1 large egg
- ¼ teaspoon salt
- ⅛ teaspoon ground nutmeg
- 4 quarts water

Method

1. Place a pot with a little bit of water on the stove to boil.
2. Peel, wash, and cube the potatoes.
3. Add a steamer basket or collider to the pot and add the potatoes. Steam for about 20 minutes or until they are tender.
4. Once cooked, remove from the pot and allow it to cool completely.
5. Place the potatoes in a potato ricer and force them through in batches. If you don't have a ricer, you can mash the potatoes. Make sure you do not over-mash, otherwise the gnocchi will be too pasty.
6. Add 3 tablespoons of flour, egg, salt, and nutmeg to the potatoes. Mix together with a fork. It should have a crumbly consistency.
7. Add in 2 more tablespoons of flour and mix. Until well combined
8. Knead the dough. Once all the flour is incorporated, stop kneading.
9. Sprinkle the last of the flour onto the work surface and place the dough on it.
10. Cut the dough in half and work with one half at a time.

11. Roll each of the pieces into a long, thin sausage shape. It should be about the width of your thumb.
12. Cut out ½ inch pieces of the dough. You should get about 20 pieces in all. Make ridges of the gnocchi by lightly pressing a fork against it.
13. Place a pot of water onto the stove to boil.
14. Once the water is boiling, add the gnocchi. Don't overcrowd the pot.
15. As they float to the top of the water you can take them out. The floating means they are fully cooked.
16. Drain and serve with your favorite sauce.

There is nothing more comforting than a big bowl of soup or stew, especially on a cold day. Soups also keep really well so you can make very large batches and save them in the fridge and the freezer for later days. You can eat these on their own or swerve with some crispy bread.

Soups and stews are also really versatile, so feel free to add your favorite ingredients. They take some time to cook but this is not time that you have to physically watch it. You can put it on and come back and check it every so often. If you have a slow cooker this is even better. You can throw all the ingredients in the pot and leave it for hours without getting involved.

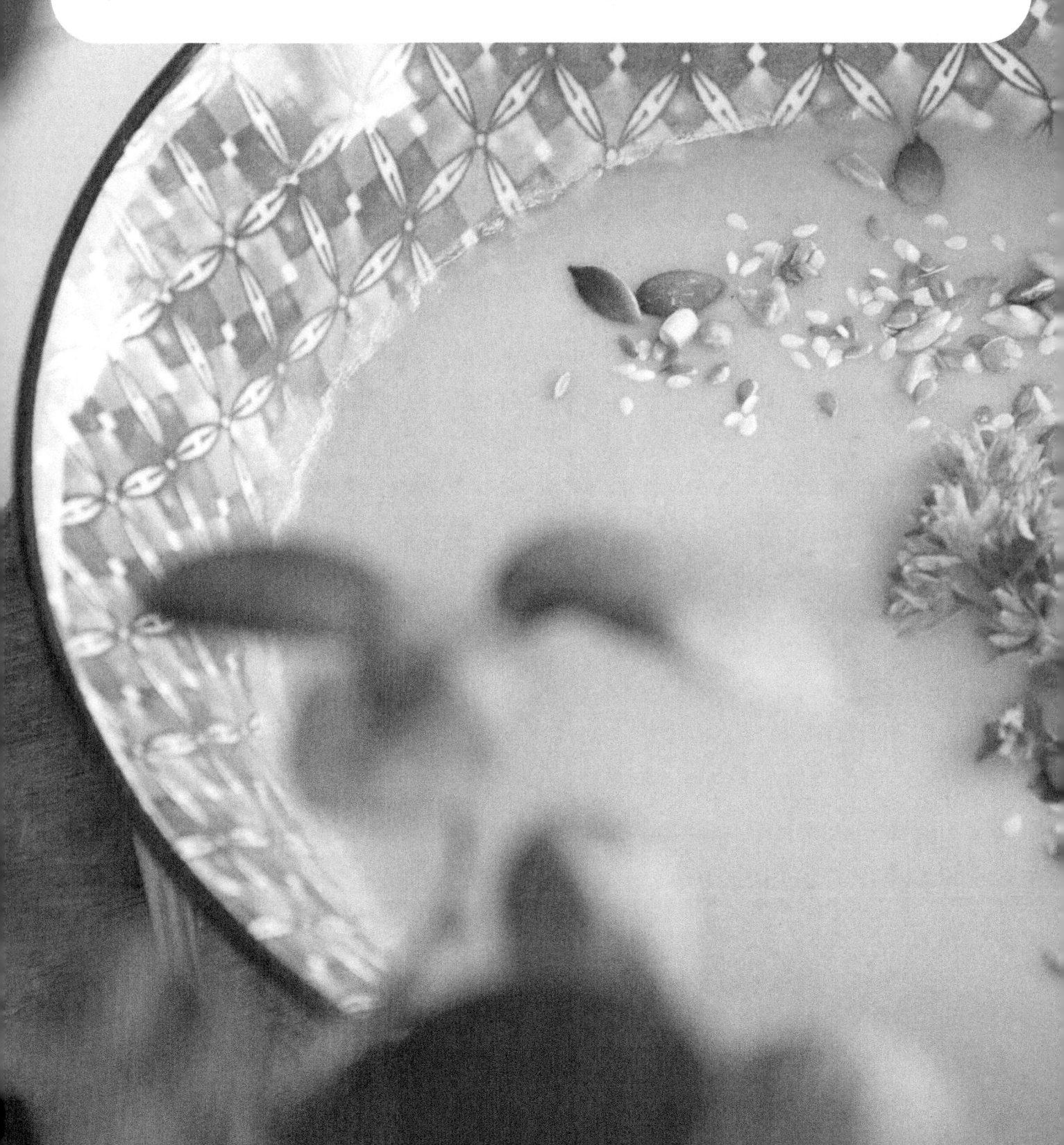

Soups and Stew

Chicken Noodle Soup — 134

Eggplant Soup — VEGETARIAN GLUTEN-FREE 135

Chicken and Barley Stew — GLUTEN-FREE 136

Chicken and Black-Eyes Pea Soup — GLUTEN-FREE 137

Chickpea and Lentil Soup — VEGAN GLUTEN-FREE 138

Turkey White Bean Soup — GLUTEN-FREE 139

Butternut Soup — VEGAN GLUTEN-FREE 140

Chicken Noodle Soup

Cal 368	**Difficulty:** Easy **Preparation time:** 15 minutes **Cook time:** 55 minutes **Servings:** 6

Nutrition per serving (g)

Fat	Saturates	Carbs	Sugars	Protein
6	2	42	6	31

Ingredients

- 2 teaspoons olive oil
- 1 lb boneless skinless chicken thighs, cut into 1-inch cubes
- onion powder, to taste
- 3 ribs celery, sliced
- 3 medium carrots, peeled and sliced
- 2 cups low sodium chicken broth
- ¼ teaspoon salt
- ½ teaspoon dried tarragon
- 4 quarts water
- 6 oz egg noodles
- 2 tablespoons fresh parsley, coarsely chopped

Method

1. Place a teaspoon of oil in a hot pot, followed by the chicken. Let it brown.
2. Add the celery and the rest of the oil, if needed. Cook for 3 minutes.
3. Add in the carrots, chicken stock, salt, tarragon, onion powder, and 4 cups of water.
4. Lower the heat and let it simmer for 45 minutes.
5. Cook the noodles in a separate pot, according to the package instructions. Drain.
6. Once everything is done, place the noodles in the bottom a bowl and pour over the soup. Serve.

Eggplant Soup

Cal 101

VEGETARIAN
GLUTEN-FREE

Difficulty: Easy
Preparation time: 20 minutes
Cook time: 100 minutes
Servings: 6

Nutrition per serving (g)

Fat	Saturates	Carbs	Sugars	Protein
1	1	18	5	5

Ingredients

- 2 cups red bell pepper, chopped
- 1 ½ lbs eggplant, quartered lengthwise
- ½ lb shallots, peeled and halved
- ½ teaspoon garlic powder
- 1 tablespoon apple cider vinegar
- Spray olive oil
- 1 teaspoon dried thyme
- 3 ½ cups low sodium vegetable broth
- ½ cup white wine
- 2 cups water
- ¼ teaspoon salt
- 1 cup skimmed milk (or milk of choice)

Method

1. Heat your oven to 400 degrees Fahrenheit.
2. Place all your vegetables on a large roasting pan and drizzle or spray olive oil on top.
3. Roast the vegetables for about 45 minutes. They should be tender and be browned in some spots.
4. Once done, remove them from the oven and let them cool.
5. Once cooled, scoop out the flesh from the eggplant. You can throw away the skin.
6. Add all the vegetables to a large pot along with the vegetable stock.
7. Place it on the heat and let it simmer for another 45 minutes.
8. Switch the heat off and let it cool down for about 10 minutes.
9. Use a stick blender to blend the contents of the pot. Add salt to taste.
10. Once smooth, place it back on the heat and add the milk.
11. Stir everything together and once it has heated through, it is ready to serve.

Chicken and Barley Stew

Cal 150
GLUTEN-FREE

Difficulty: Easy
Preparation time: 10 minutes
Cook time: 5 to 6 hours
Servings: 6

Nutrition per serving (g)

Fat	Saturates	Carbs	Sugars	Protein
3.3	1.5	32.1	1.7	24.3

Ingredients

- 2 chicken breasts
- ¾ cup of barley
- 48 oz low-sodium chicken broth
- 1, 16 oz. bag frozen mixed vegetables
- ¼ teaspoon of garlic powder*
- ¼ teaspoon onion powder*
- 2 teaspoons Italian seasoning (or a mix of herbs like basil, oregano, and thyme)
- 2 bay leaves
- Salt
- 2 cups chopped baby spinach

Method

1. Throw all the ingredients, except the spinach, into a slow cooker or crockpot.
2. Let it cook on a low setting, with the lid on, for 5 to 6 hours.
3. Add in the spinach when the stew has about 30 minutes left to cook.
4. Remove the bay leaves and throw them away.
5. Remove the chicken and shred it. Place it back into the stew and mix it all together.
6. Serve hot.

If the onion and garlic powder triggers acid reflux you can add less of it or you could just omit both onion and garlic powder completely.

Chicken and Black-Eyes Pea Soup

Cal 360
GLUTEN-FREE

Difficulty: Easy
Preparation time: 15 minutes
Cook time: 55 minutes
Servings: 4

Nutrition per serving (g)

Fat	Saturates	Carbs	Sugars	Protein
8	2	37	7	38

Ingredients

- 1 teaspoon olive oil
- ½ teaspoon onion powder
- 2 ribs celery, diced
- 1 lb boneless skinless chicken thighs, cut into 1-inch cubes
- 2 teaspoon dried sage
- ½ teaspoon dried thyme
- ½ teaspoon salt
- 3 cups low sodium chicken broth
- 2 cups water
- 2, 15 oz can no salt added blackeyed peas, drained
- 8 oz fresh spinach

Method

1. Heat up a large pot or saucepan.
2. Add in the oil and celery. Cook this down for about 6 minutes.
3. Once it has begun to soften, add the chicken, sage, onion powder and thyme.
4. Cook for another 6 minutes, letting the chicken brown. Stir occasionally to prevent the chicken from sticking to the pan.
5. Pour in the broth, water, blackeyed peas, and salt.
6. Let the soup simmer for about 40 minutes. Stir occasionally.
7. Once the soup is ready, place a few handfuls of spinach at the bottom of a bowl and pour the soup over.

Chickpea and Lentil Soup

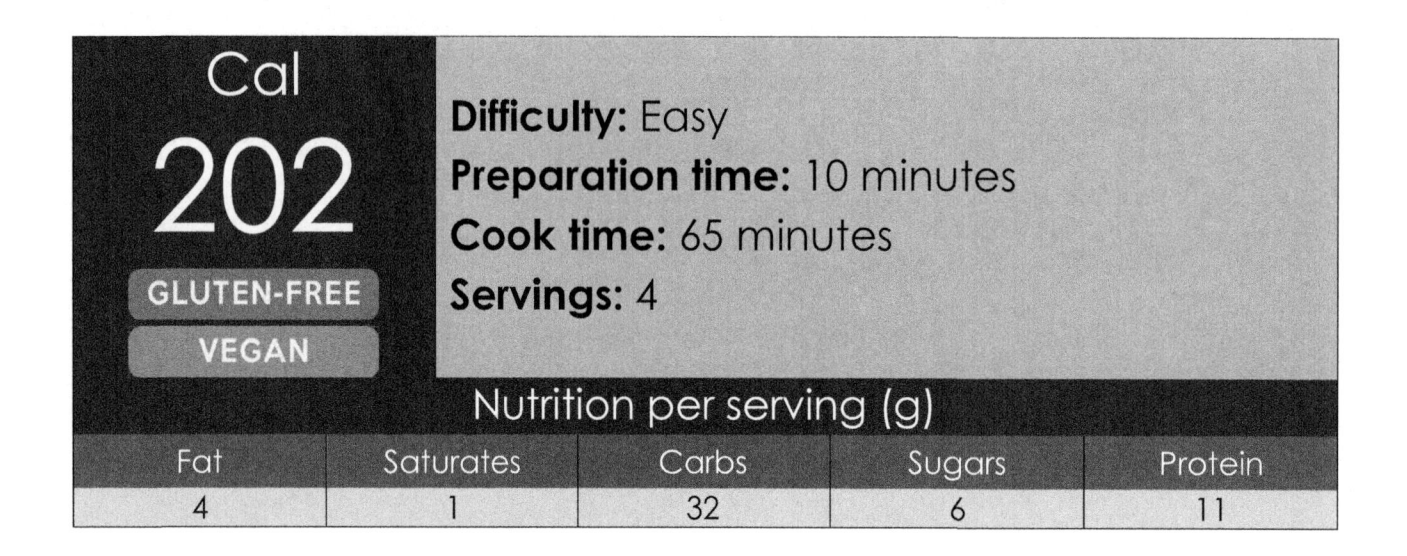

Cal 202

GLUTEN-FREE
VEGAN

Difficulty: Easy
Preparation time: 10 minutes
Cook time: 65 minutes
Servings: 4

Nutrition per serving (g)

Fat	Saturates	Carbs	Sugars	Protein
4	1	32	6	11

Ingredients

- 2 quarts water
- 4 oz dried lentils
- 4 oz dried chickpeas
- 2 teaspoons olive oil
- 4 oz celery, diced
- 4 oz carrots, peeled and diced
- 3 cups no salt added vegetable stock
- 1 cup water
- ¼ teaspoon salt
- 3 bay leaves

Method

1. Pour the lentils, chickpeas, and water into a bowl. Let it stand overnight or for at least 10 hours.
2. Once they are done soaking, drain, and set aside.
3. Place a saucepan on the heat and add in some oil.
4. Add the celery and cook until translucent.
5. Next, add in the carrots and cook for about 3 minutes.
6. Pour in the vegetable stock, water, bay leaves, chickpeas, and lentils.
7. Let simmer for about 45 minutes.
8. Add in some salt and allow it to simmer for a further 15 minutes.
9. Pour into bowls to serve.

Turkey White Bean Soup

Cal 338
GLUTEN-FREE

Difficulty: Easy
Preparation time: 15 minutes
Cook time: 120 minutes
Servings: 8

Nutrition per serving (g)

Fat	Saturates	Carbs	Sugars	Protein
5	2	29	2	42

Ingredients

- 2 quarts water
- Leftover turkey bones*
- 2 lbs leftover turkey meat
- 3, 15 oz can no salt added white beans, drained and rinsed
- 3 large ribs celery, thickly sliced
- 3 large carrots, peeled and cut into large chunks
- ¾ teaspoons salt
- 1 tablespoon dried sage

Method

1. Place a large pot on the stove and pour in the water.
2. Add the turkey bones and let it simmer for 30 minutes
3. Stain and throw away the bones.
4. Pour the broth into a pot with the turkey meat, white beans, celery, carrots, salt, and sage.
5. Let the soup simmer for 90 minutes.
6. Serve in bowls when ready.

If you do not have any leftover turkey then cook the turkey and then continue with the rest of the steps.

Butternut Soup

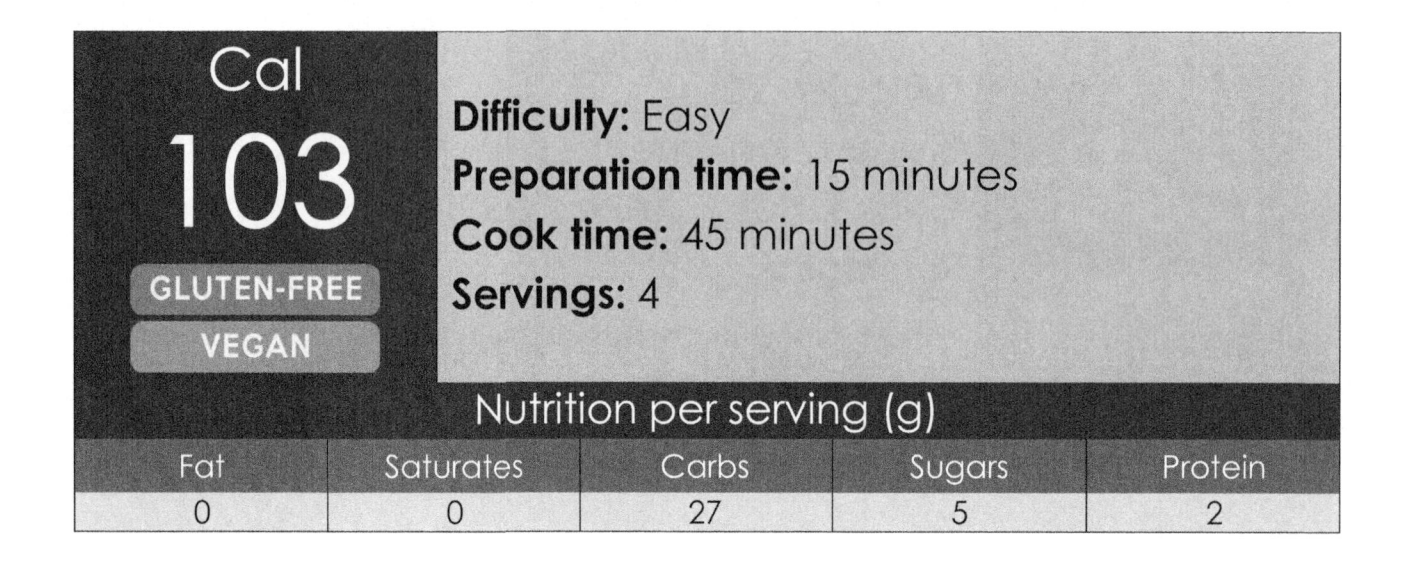

Cal 103

GLUTEN-FREE
VEGAN

Difficulty: Easy
Preparation time: 15 minutes
Cook time: 45 minutes
Servings: 4

Nutrition per serving (g)

Fat	Saturates	Carbs	Sugars	Protein
0	0	27	5	2

Ingredients

- 2 cups water
- 2 lbs butternut squash
- ½ teaspoon salt
- ½ teaspoon dried thyme leaves
- ⅛ teaspoon ground nutmeg
- 1 cup water

Method

1. Cut up your butternut into even-sized cubes.
2. Place the butternut in a steamer and let it cook for about 30 minutes.
3. If you do not have a steamer or a steamer basket you can use a colander placed inside a pot with a little bit of water.
4. Once the squash is nice and tender set it aside to cool.
5. Once cooled add the butternut to a pot with a bit of water.
6. Use a stick blender to puree the squash until it is smooth.
7. Place the soup on the stove to heat up. If it is too thick add some more water.
8. Stir in the nutmeg, thyme, and salt.
9. Keep adding water until it is your desired consistency.
10. Once you are happy, serve in bowls.

Sometimes we all need a little extra in life. These are great little things that you can make for various situations. They are generally very easy to make and are definitely delicious.

Snacks, Sides, and Extras

Low Acid Tomato Sauce	VEGAN	GLUTEN-FREE	144
Basil Pesto	VEGETARIAN		145
Dill Oil	VEGAN		146
Ginger Mashed Potatoes	VEGETARIAN		147
Baked French Fries	VEGAN		148
Bok Choy Slaw	VEGAN		149
Parsnip French Fries	VEGAN		150
Stuffed Mushroom Caps			151
Sautéed Spinach with Apples and Walnuts	VEGAN		152
Crispy Quinoa	VEGAN		153
Artichoke and Spinach Dip	VEGETARIAN		154
Olive, Walnut, and Edamame Mix	VEGAN		155
Candied Pecans	VEGAN		156
Dried Persimmon	VEGAN		157
Ginger Tea	VEGAN	GLUTEN-FREE	158

Low Acid GERD-Friendly Tomato Sauce*

Cal 46

GLUTEN-FREE
VEGAN

Difficulty: Easy
Preparation time: 5 minutes
Cook time: 190 minutes
Servings: 10

Nutrition per serving (g)

Fat	Saturates	Carbs	Sugars	Protein
2	0	8	4	1

Ingredients

- 1 tablespoon olive oil
- ¼ teaspoon onion powder
- ¼ teaspoon garlic powder
- 2, 28-oz. cans no salt added diced tomatoes
- 3 cups water
- 1 ½ teaspoons baking soda

Method

1. Pour the oil into a large pot and place it on the heat.
2. Add the onion and garlic powder and let fry in the oil for about a minute.
3. Pour in the water and tomatoes. Reduce the heat to low.
4. Let this cook for about 3 hours, stirring occasionally. Add a bit more water if you see it getting too thick.
5. Remove the pot from the heat and let it cook for about 10 minutes.
6. Add in the baking soda about a half teaspoon at a time. Stir and let it bubble.
7. Once it stops bubbling, add another bit of baking soda. Stir and repeat the steps until all the baking soda has been used.
8. Stir every few minutes until the sauce is no longer bubbling.
9. Serve or let it cool and store in the fridge or freezer.

You can use this recipe for other recipes that call for a tomato sauce or canned tomatoes or you can just enjoy it over pasta.

Basil Pesto

Cal 86 — VEGETARIAN

Difficulty: Easy
Preparation time: 5 minutes
Cook time: 0 minutes
Servings: 6

Nutrition per serving (g)

Fat	Saturates	Carbs	Sugars	Protein
8	2	2	0	3

Ingredients

- 2 tablespoons pine nuts
- Garlic powder, to taste
- 4 cups fresh basil
- 1 oz Parmigiano-Reggiano, grated
- 2 tablespoon water
- 1 tablespoon white wine vinegar
- 2 tablespoons extra virgin olive oil

Method

1. Place all the ingredients into a food processor or blender.
2. Pulse until smooth.
3. Keep in the fridge until ready to serve.

Dill Oil

Cal 40

VEGAN

Difficulty: Easy
Preparation time: 5 minutes
Cook time: 5 minutes
Servings: 8

Nutrition per serving (g)

Fat	Saturates	Carbs	Sugars	Protein
5	1	0	0	3

Ingredients

- ¼ cup extra virgin olive oil
- ½ cup fresh dill leaves

Method

1. Place the oil on the stove to just heat through.
2. Once warm, switch off the heat and add the dill leaves.
3. Let stand for 20 minutes.
4. Pour into a blender and blend until smooth.

You can do this with other herbs to make delicious infused oils for kinds of pasta, soups, and salads.

Ginger Mashed Potatoes

Cal 107
VEGETARIAN

Difficulty: Easy
Preparation time: 15 minutes
Cook time: 20 minutes
Servings: 4

Nutrition per serving (g)

Fat	Saturates	Carbs	Sugars	Protein
2	1	20	3	4

Ingredients

- 2 quarts water
- 1 lb Yukon Gold potatoes, cubed
- 1 teaspoon unsalted butter
- ⅓ cup nonfat buttermilk
- ⅓ cup milk of choice
- ¼ teaspoon salt
- 1 tablespoon fresh ginger

Method

1. Place the water on to boil and then add the potatoes.
2. Let the potatoes simmer for about 20 minutes or until soft.
3. Drain and pour in the rest of the ingredients.
4. Mash until they are as smooth as you would like.
5. Serve.

Baked French Fries

Cal 194

VEGAN

Difficulty: Easy
Preparation time: 10 minutes
Cook time: 40 minutes
Servings: 4

Nutrition per serving (g)

Fat	Saturates	Carbs	Sugars	Protein
4	1	37	2	4

Ingredients

- 4 medium russet potatoes
- 1 tablespoon olive oil
- ½ teaspoon kosher salt

Method

1. Preheat the oven to 400 degrees Fahrenheit.
2. Line a baking sheet with some parchment paper.
3. Wash the potatoes to remove any dirt.
4. Slice the potatoes into large slices so that you have evenly sized fries.
5. Place the fries onto the baking sheets.
6. Drizzle with olive oil and sprinkle over salt.
7. Toss and place in the oven.
8. Allow to bake for about 40 minutes. Toss a few times during cooking.
9. Once golden, remove from the oven and place aside to cool.

Bok Choy Slaw

Cal 51

VEGAN

Difficulty: Easy
Preparation time: 10 minutes
Cook time: 0 minutes
Servings: 2

Nutrition per serving (g)

Fat	Saturates	Carbs	Sugars	Protein
3	0.5	4	2	2

Ingredients

- 8 oz bok choy, thinly sliced
- ¼ cup fresh basil leaves, chiffonade
- 2 teaspoons dark sesame oil
- 1 teaspoon rice vinegar
- 2 teaspoons low sodium soy sauce or tamari sauce
- ½ teaspoon sugar
- 1 teaspoon white or black sesame seeds

Method

1. Toss all the ingredients together in a mixing bowl.
2. Allow to stand for a few minutes before serving.

Parsnip French Fries

Cal 95

VEGAN

Difficulty: Easy
Preparation time: 10 minutes
Cook time: 25 minutes
Servings: 4

Nutrition per serving (g)

Fat	Saturates	Carbs	Sugars	Protein
1.5	0	20	6	2

Ingredients

- 1 lb parsnips
- 1 quart cold water
- 1 tray ice cubes
- ⅛ teaspoon salt
- ⅛ teaspoon dried rosemary
- Spray olive oil

Method

1. Cut the parsnips into french fries.
2. Place them in a bowl filled with cold water and ice cubes. Leave them to soak for 30 minutes.
3. Drain and pat them dry.
4. Preheat the oven to 400 degrees Fahrenheit.
5. Place the parsnips in a bowl and spray with oil. Sprinkle over the salt and rosemary.
6. Pour the fries onto a baking tray and bake for 25 minutes.
7. Turn them about 3 times through the cooking process.
8. Remove and serve while hot.

Stuffed Mushroom Caps

Cal 105	Difficulty: Easy Preparation time: 10 minutes Cook time: 25 minutes Servings: 8

Nutrition per serving (g)

Fat	Saturates	Carbs	Sugars	Protein
7	3	6	1	5

Ingredients

- ¼ of garlic powder
- ½ cup breadcrumbs
- 6 slices turkey bacon, baked until crispy and crumbled
- 5 oz spinach chopped
- ¼ gruyere, grated
- ¼ romano, grated
- 24 medium mushrooms, stems removed
- ¼ olive oil

Method

1. Preheat the oven to 375 degrees Fahrenheit.
2. Place the mushroom caps on a greased baking tray and bake for 10 minutes.
3. Cook mushroom stems, and turkey bacon in a pan with a bit of oil then add the garlic powder.
4. Add the spinach and cook until wilted.
5. Add the breadcrumbs and cheese.
6. Remove the caps from the oven and fill them with the mixture.
7. Place them back in the oven to bake for 15 minutes.
8. Serve.

Sautéed Spinach with Apples and Walnuts

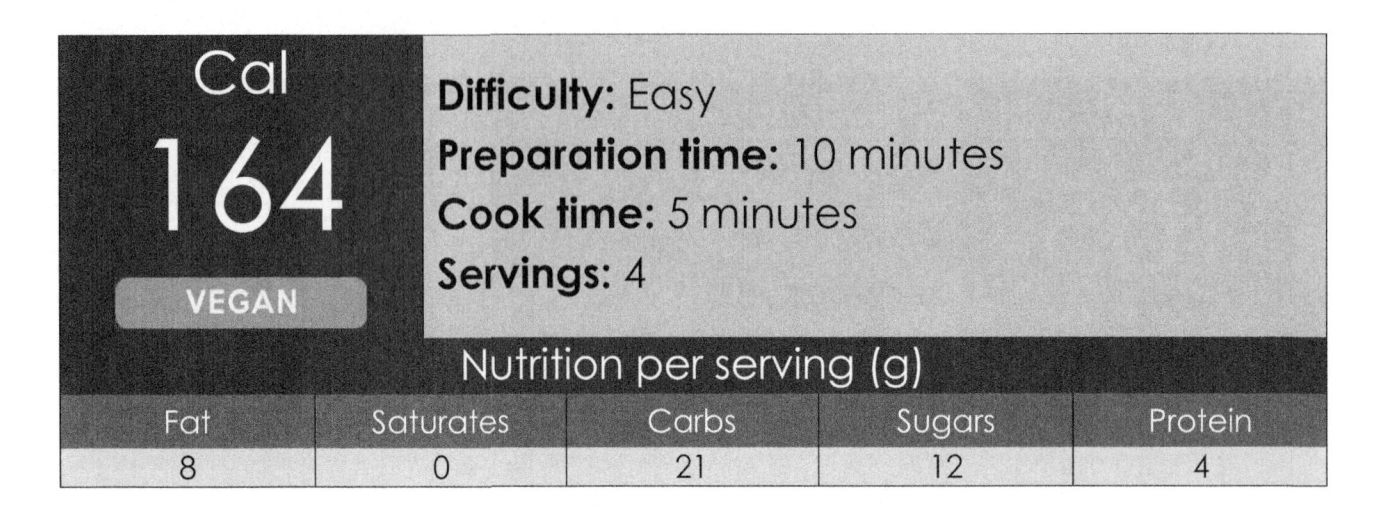

Cal 164

VEGAN

Difficulty: Easy
Preparation time: 10 minutes
Cook time: 5 minutes
Servings: 4

Nutrition per serving (g)

Fat	Saturates	Carbs	Sugars	Protein
8	0	21	12	4

Ingredients

- 1 tablespoon olive oil
- ¼ cup walnut pieces
- 1 large apple (diced)
- ¼ cup raisins
- 1 lb fresh spinach
- ¼ teaspoon salt

Method

1. Place a nonstick pan on the heat and add in the olive oil.
2. Add the walnuts and toast for a minute.
3. Pour in the apples and raisins and allow them to cook for abotu2 minutes.
4. Add in the spinach and wilt. Sprinkle in salt.
5. Switch off the heat and serve as a side.

Crispy Quinoa

Cal 38
VEGAN

Difficulty: Easy
Preparation time: 0 minutes
Cook time: 45 minutes
Servings: 6

Nutrition per serving (g)

Fat	Saturates	Carbs	Sugars	Protein
1	0	7	0	1

Ingredients

- 2 cups water
- ½ cup quinoa
- ¼ teaspoon salt

Method

1. Place water on to boil in a saucepan.
2. Pour in the quinoa and the salt and let cook until the water has evaporated.
3. Switch off the stove, place the lid on, and allow to rest for about 5 minutes.
4. Pour the cooked quinoa onto a baking sheet and allow it to dry completely for 2 hours.
5. Preheat the oven to 325 degrees Fahrenheit.
6. Place the quinoa in the oven and let toast for 30 minutes.
7. Gently stir every 10 minutes or so.
8. Once toasted, remove from the oven and allow to cool.
9. Place in an airtight container.
10. You can use it as a topping for fish, soups, and salads.

Artichoke and Spinach Dip

Cal 41

VEGETARIAN

Difficulty: Easy
Preparation time: 10 minutes
Cook time: 5 minutes
Servings: 16

Nutrition per serving (g)

Fat	Saturates	Carbs	Sugars	Protein
2	1	5	1	3

Ingredients

- 2, 15 oz cans artichoke hearts, packed in water
- 2, 10 oz packages frozen spinach, thawed
- ½ cup fat-free mayonnaise
- 2 ½ oz mozzarella cheese, grated
- 1 oz reduced-fat cream cheese
- ¼ teaspoon salt
- ⅛ teaspoon ground nutmeg

Method

1. Thaw out the spinach and then drain it.
2. Place it in a sieve and press out all the excess water. Reserve this water for later.
3. Brain the artichokes and place them in a food processor, along with the spinach, mozzarella, cream cheese, salt, nutmeg, and mayonnaise.
4. Process until the mixture is smooth. Ad in a few tablespoons of the spinach water to help achieve a smooth texture. You should only need about 2 spoon fulls.
5. When you are ready to serve the dip, microwave it to melt the cheese.
6. Microwave 30 seconds at a time until it has fully melted. Stir between each interval. Do not overcook. Serve immediately.

Olive, Walnut, and Edamame Mix

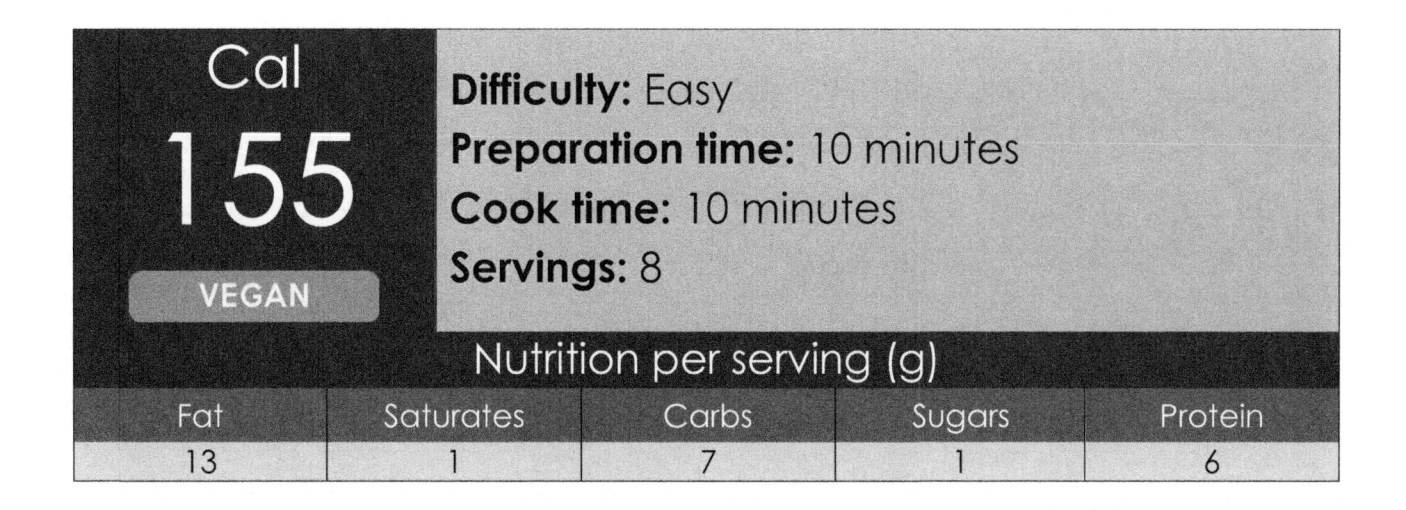

Cal **155**

VEGAN

Difficulty: Easy
Preparation time: 10 minutes
Cook time: 10 minutes
Servings: 8

Nutrition per serving (g)

Fat	Saturates	Carbs	Sugars	Protein
13	1	7	1	6

Ingredients

- 1 cup walnuts, toasted
- 1 cup Kalamata olives, pitted
- 2 cups frozen shelled edamame, defrosted
- 1 teaspoon extra-virgin olive oil
- ½ teaspoon garlic powder
- 1 tablespoon fresh rosemary leaves

Method

1. Place all the ingredients into a large bowl.
2. Toss and serve.
3. If there are any leftovers, place in an airtight container and in the refrigerator.

Candied Pecans

Cal 95

VEGAN

Difficulty: Easy
Preparation time: 0 minutes
Cook time: 15 minutes
Servings: 4

Nutrition per serving (g)

Fat	Saturates	Carbs	Sugars	Protein
10	1	2	1	1

Ingredients

- ½ cup pecan pieces
- 1/16 teaspoon salt
- 2 teaspoon maple syrup

Method

1. Place a nonstick pan on the stove and heat up to medium heat.
2. Toast the pecans for a few minutes then sprinkle in the salt.
3. Pour in the maple syrup and let bubble for a few seconds.
4. Shake the pan to coat the pecans.
5. Remove from the heat and stir.
6. Pour out the pecans on some parchment paper and separate the pecans before they dry.
7. Once dried, you can use them as a garnish for desserts or breakfasts. You could just enjoy them as a snack.

Dried Persimmon

Cal 188

VEGAN

Difficulty: Easy
Preparation time: 5 minutes
Cook time: 120 minutes
Servings: 6

Nutrition per serving (g)

Fat	Saturates	Carbs	Sugars	Protein
0	0	31	21	1

Ingredients

- 6 medium Fuyu persimmons

Method

1. Preheat oven to 250 degrees Fahrenheit
2. Slice the persimmons into ¼ inch thick rounds.
3. Place the rounds on a wire rack, making sure that they are not overlapping.
4. Place in the oven and bake for 90 to 120 minutes. The centers should be dry and the edges will be curling up.

Ginger Tea

Cal 2

VEGAN
GLUTEN-FREE

Difficulty: Easy
Preparation time: 5 minutes
Cook time: 5 minutes
Servings: 1

Nutrition per serving (g)

Fat	Saturates	Carbs	Sugars	Protein
0	0	0	0	0

Ingredients

- 1-inch chunk of fresh ginger, sliced into pieces no wider than ¼-inch
- 1 cup water

Method

1. Place a pan on the heat and all the water and ginger pieces.
2. Let simmer for 5 to 10 minutes, depending on how strong you want the ginger to be.
3. If it ends up being too strong just add more water.
4. Pour into a mug. Serve.
5. Add some sweetener if desired, honey or maple syrup are great choices.

This one is for all the people out there with a sweet tooth. I could not create a recipe book and not add in some delicious desserts. A nice sweet treat is a perfect way to end a meal or the day. There is a misconception that desserts have to be unhealthy but that cannot be further from the truth. Many of these desserts are healthy, nutritious, and delicious. There are some more indulgent options for special occasions. It is important that you enjoy the food you make. Try out these desserts to kill you sweet cravings the right way.

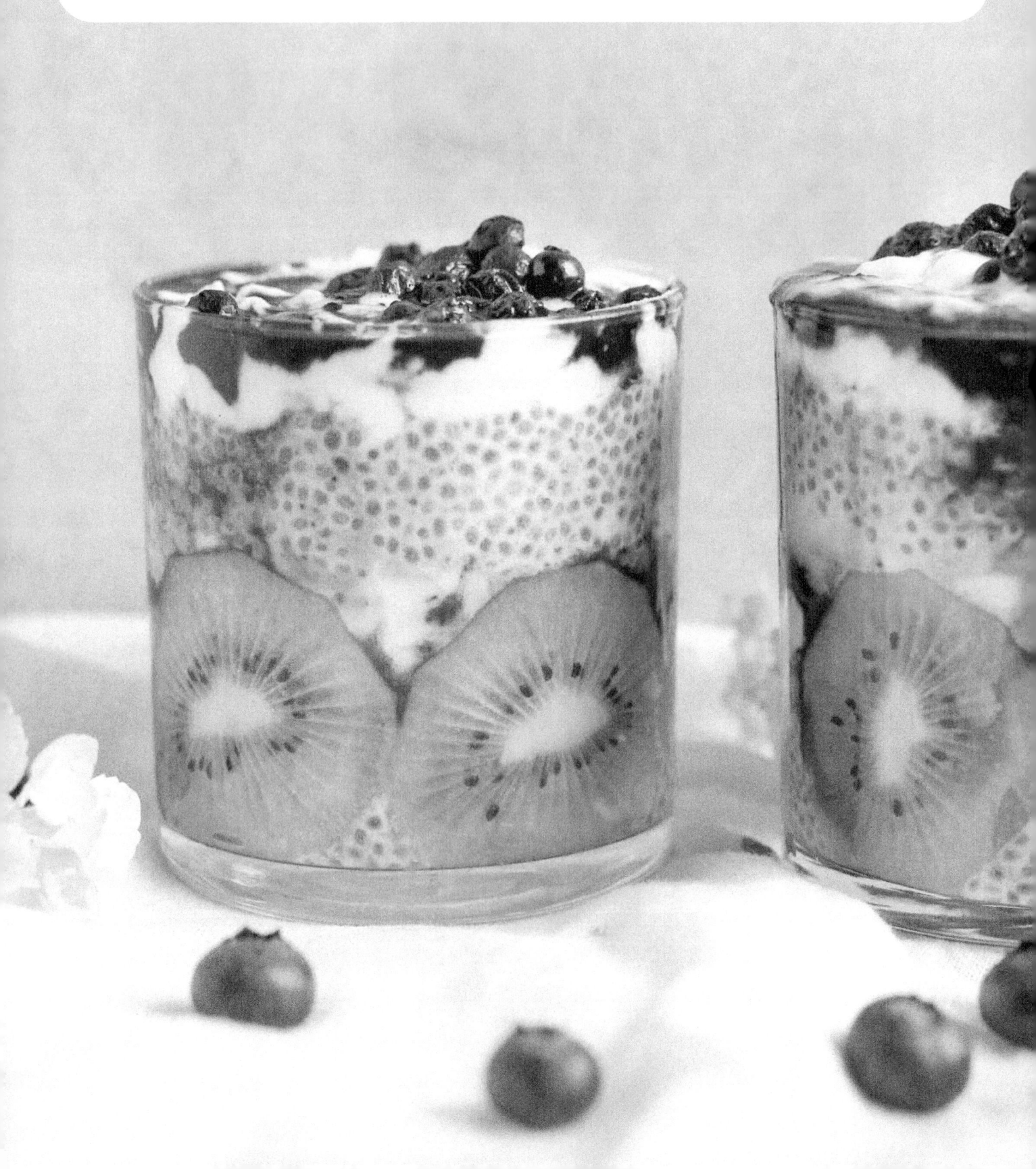

Desserts

Healthy Apple Crisp	VEGETARIAN	162
Vanilla Almond Parfait	VEGETARIAN	163
Coconut rice pudding	VEGETARIAN	164
Chia Pudding With Honeydew Melon	VEGAN	165
Blueberry and Banana Sorbet	VEGAN	166
Watermelon Parfait	VEGETARIAN	167
Strawberry Sorbet	VEGAN GLUTEN-FREE	168
Angel Food Cupcakes	VEGETARIAN	169
Crème Brûlée	VEGETARIAN	170
Arroz con Leche	VEGETARIAN	172
Flan	VEGETARIAN GLUTEN-FREE	174
Sweet Potato Tarts	VEGETARIAN	176
Papaya, Yogurt and Walnut Boat	VEGETARIAN	178

Healthy Apple Crisp

Cal 195

VEGETARIAN

Difficulty: Normal
Preparation time: 25 minutes
Cook time: 30 minutes
Servings: 6

Nutrition per serving (g)

Fat	Saturates	Carbs	Sugars	Protein
10	4	28	17	2

Ingredients

- 4 medium apples, peeled, seeded, and diced
- 1 teaspoon cornstarch
- 1 teaspoon cinnamon
- 1 teaspoon cream of tartar mix in ¼ cup of water
- ½ teaspoon lemongrass, finely chopped
- 2 tablespoons sugar
- 3 tablespoons unsalted butter, cold, diced into small pieces
- 2 tablespoons all-purpose flour
- ½ cup rolled oats
- 2 tablespoons light brown sugar, packed
- ½ teaspoon kosher salt
- ⅓ cup chopped walnuts
- 6 tablespoons 100% apple juice

Method

1. Preheat the oven to 350 degrees Fahrenheit.
2. Spray 6 ramekins with cooking spray. Set aside.
3. Mix together the apples, cornstarch, cinnamon, lemongrass, cream of tartar mixture, and sugar.
4. Set it aside for a few minutes.
5. In another bowl, stir the butter, flour, oats, brown sugar, salt, and walnuts. This is the topping.
6. Spoon the apple mixture into the ramekins and then pour over the topping.
7. Pour a tablespoon of apple juice over each one.
8. Place the ramekins on a baking sheet and bake in the oven for about 30 minutes. The top should be golden brown.
9. Remove from the oven and let cook for a few minutes before serving.

Vanilla Almond Parfait

Cal 199

VEGETARIAN

Difficulty: Easy
Preparation time: 5 minutes
Cook time: 15 minutes
Servings: 4

Nutrition per serving (g)

Fat	Saturates	Carbs	Sugars	Protein
7	4	28	16	2

Ingredients

- 1 cup vanilla almond milk (unsweetened)
- 1 cup Greek yogurt (plain low fat)
- 2 tablespoons agave
- 1 teaspoon vanilla
- ⅛ teaspoon kosher salt
- ¼ cup chia seeds
- 2 cups sliced strawberries
- ¼ cup sliced almonds
- 4 teaspoons agave for serving

Method

1. Mix the first 5 ingredients in a bowl.
2. Stir in the chia seeds and let stand overnight.
3. Mix the strawberries, agave, and almonds together.
4. Layer the parfait and serve.

Coconut rice pudding

Cal 190
VEGETARIAN

Difficulty: Easy
Preparation time: 5 minutes
Cook time: 15 minutes
Servings: 6

Nutrition per serving (g)

Fat	Saturates	Carbs	Sugars	Protein
6	2	31	16	3

Ingredients

- 3/4 cup low-fat milk
- 1/2 cup coconut milk
- 1 large pear grated
- 2 tbs. honey
- 1 (1oz) package instant fat-free, sugar-free vanilla pudding mix
- 2 cups cooked rice
- 1/4 cup shredded coconut
- 1/2 teaspoon ground ginger

Method

1. Boil the milk, coconut milk, pear, and honey for 5 minutes.
2. Remove from the heat. Mix in the pudding, then the rice, ginger, and coconut.
3. Let mixture stand in the pot for 10 minutes before serving.

Chia Pudding With Honeydew Melon

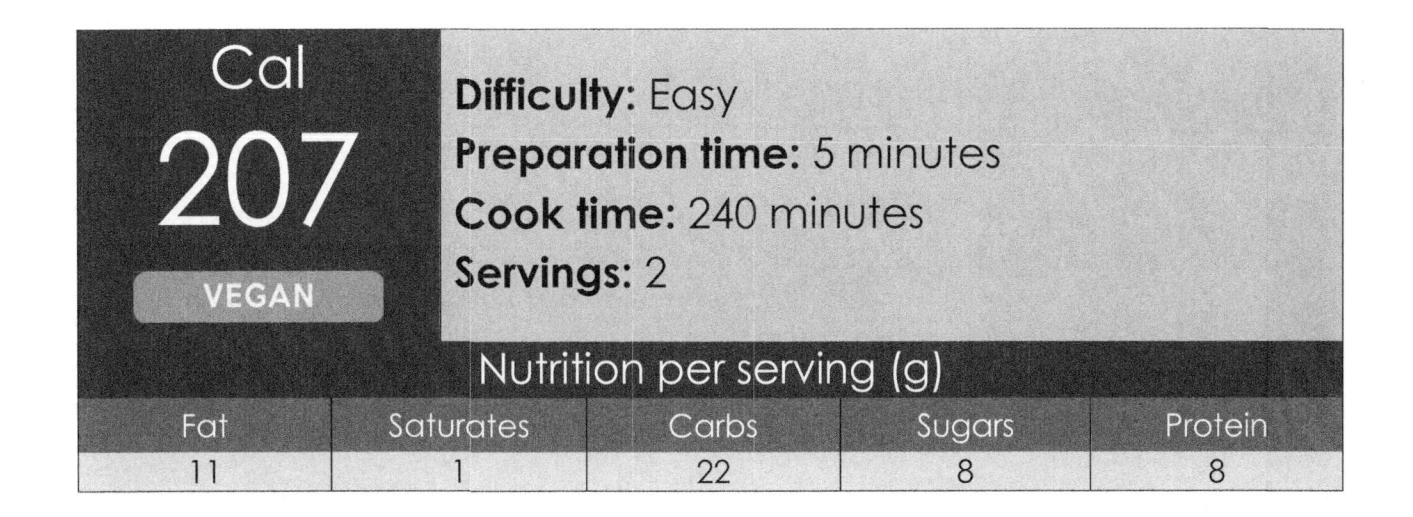

Cal 207
VEGAN

Difficulty: Easy
Preparation time: 5 minutes
Cook time: 240 minutes
Servings: 2

Nutrition per serving (g)

Fat	Saturates	Carbs	Sugars	Protein
11	1	22	8	8

Ingredients

- 1 cup vanilla soy milk
- ¼ cup chia seeds
- ½ cup finely chopped honeydew melon

Method

1. Pour the chia seeds and soy milk into a large bowl. Stir well.
2. Cover the bowl with plastic wrap and leave in the fridge for 2 hours.
3. Take it out of the fridge and mix it again.
4. Place the plastic wrap back on and leave the bowl in the fridge for another 2 hours. If you can leave it overnight, that would be ideal.
5. Spoon into separate bowls and top with the melon. Serve.

This recipe is very versatile so you can add whatever flavoring and toppings you like.

Blueberry and Banana Sorbet

Cal 229

VEGAN

Difficulty: Easy
Preparation time: 5 minutes
Cook time: 0 minutes
Servings: 2

Nutrition per serving (g)

Fat	Saturates	Carbs	Sugars	Protein
11	1	34	21	3.5

Ingredients

- 2 cup of frozen blueberries
- 2 bananas
- ¼ cup chopped walnuts

Method

1. Place the blueberries and banana into a high speed food processor.
2. Process until the mixture is smooth.
3. Spoon the mixture into two bowls.
4. Either mix in the chopped walnuts or sprinkle them over the top of the sorbet.

Watermelon Parfait

Cal 319
VEGETARIAN

Difficulty: Easy
Preparation time: 10 minutes
Cook time: 0 minutes
Servings: 4

Nutrition per serving (g)

Fat	Saturates	Carbs	Sugars	Protein
15	6	50	24	13

Ingredients

- 1 cup Cantaloupe
- 16 oz fat-free strawberry yogurt
- 2 cups low-fat granola
- 1 apple, peeled, cored, and diced
- 1 cup seedless watermelon, diced

Method

1. Layer the ingredients in glasses. ¼ cup of cantaloupe, followed by ¼ cup yogurt, then ¼ cup granola.
2. Repeat the layering again and top with the watermelon and apple.
3. Add a spoon of yogurt to the top and sprinkle with the granola.
4. Serve chilled.

Strawberry Sorbet

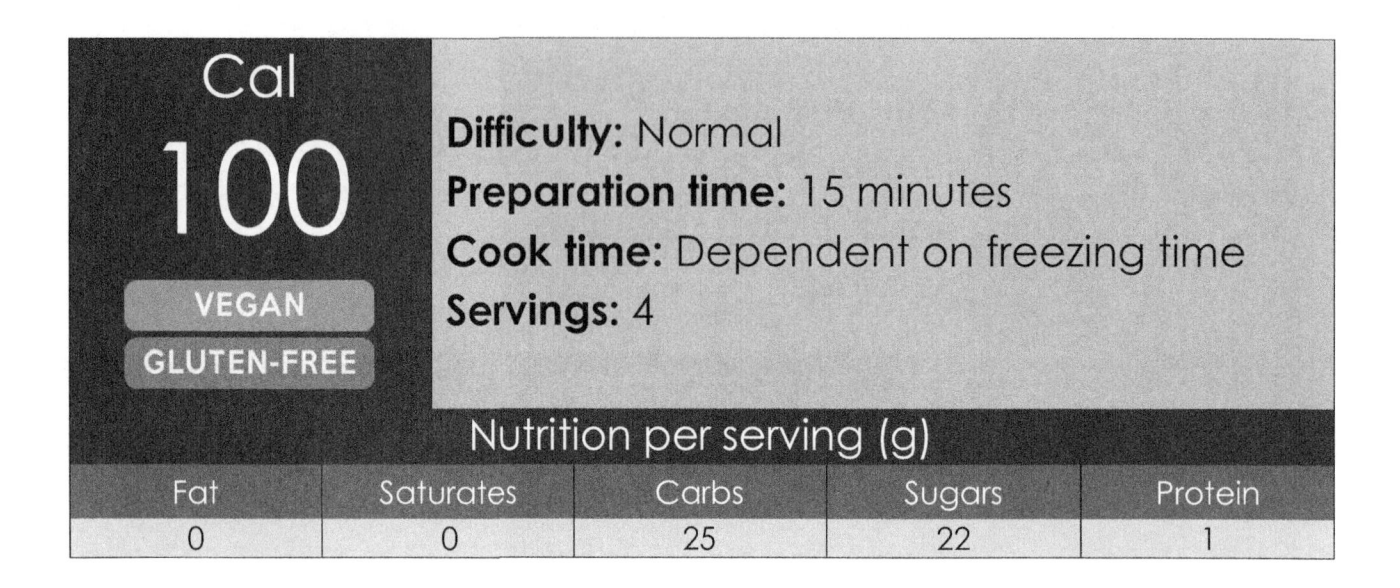

Cal 100

VEGAN
GLUTEN-FREE

Difficulty: Normal
Preparation time: 15 minutes
Cook time: Dependent on freezing time
Servings: 4

Nutrition per serving (g)

Fat	Saturates	Carbs	Sugars	Protein
0	0	25	22	1

Ingredients

- ½ cup water
- ⅓ cup sugar
- 1 lb fresh strawberries, hulled

Method

1. Pour the water and sugar into a pot and place over high heat.
2. Whisk it together until the sugar dissolves. Do this for a further minute before removing it from the heat.
3. Leave this to cool for about 5 minutes.
4. Place the strawberries and the sugar and water into a blender.
5. Pulse for about a minute or until the mixture is a smooth consistency.
6. Pour it into a storage container and place it in the freezer.
7. Take it out every 10 minutes and whisk vigorously.
8. Once the mixture begins to thicken, stop using the whisk, and start using a rubber spatula to fold the mixture.
9. Keep doing this until the mixture has reached the consistency you like.
10. Serve. You can add some fresh strawberries on top for a garnish.

Angel Food Cupcakes

Cal 72

VEGETARIAN

Difficulty: Normal
Preparation time: 20 minutes
Cook time: 15 minutes
Servings: 12

Nutrition per serving (g)

Fat	Saturates	Carbs	Sugars	Protein
0	0	15	11	2

Ingredients

- ½ cup cake flour
- ¼ cup powdered sugar
- ¼ teaspoon kosher salt
- 6 large egg whites (room temperature)
- ½ teaspoon cream of tartar
- 1 teaspoon vanilla extract
- ½ cup granulated sugar

Method

1. Preheat the oven to 350 degrees Fahrenheit.
2. Place cupcake liners inside a cupcake tin and set aside for later.
3. Sift cake flour, powdered sugar, and salt into a bowl.
4. Take out a small bowl and pour in the egg whites. Beat until they start frothing.
5. Add the cream of tartar and the vanilla. Beat with an electric mixer until it forms stiff peaks.
6. Pour in the sugar while you continue beating the mixture.
7. Once the sugar is all mixed in you can switch off the mixer.

Crème Brûlée

Cal 161
VEGETARIAN

Difficulty: Normal
Preparation time: 5 minutes
Cook time: 90 minutes
Servings: 4

Nutrition per serving (g)

Fat	Saturates	Carbs	Sugars	Protein
5	2	20	19	9

Ingredients

- 2 cups 2% milk
- ½ cup nonfat dry milk powder
- 1 teaspoon pure vanilla extract
- 3 tablespoons granulated sugar
- ⅛ teaspoon salt
- 2 large egg yolks
- 8 teaspoons granulated sugar

Method

1. Place the 2% milk, dry milk powder, and vanilla extract in a pot and place it on the heat.

2. Stir continuously and make sure it does not boil. Just before it reaches boiling, switch off the heat.

3. Let cool overnight in the fridge.

4. When you are ready to make the Crème Brûlée, preheat the oven to 300 degrees Fahrenheit.

5. Place the ramekins you will be using in a roasting dish. Pour water in the dish until it reaches ⅔ up the outside of the ramekins.

6. Take the ramekins out of the water bath and place the roasting dish with the water in the oven.

7. Let the water heat up for about 20 minutes.

8. Get out a bowl and place the sugar, egg yolks, and salt in it. Cream together.

9. Strain the cooled milk mixture into the egg mixture.

10. Whisk until well blended.

11. Pour the mixture into the ramekins and place them in the water bath in the oven.

12. Let it cook for 60 minutes.

13. Pull it out of the oven and let it cool for 30 minutes in the water bath.

14. Cover with plastic wrap and place in the fridge overnight.

15. When you are ready to serve it, pour about 2 teaspoons of sugar on each dessert.

16. Use a blowtorch to melt the sugar. Tilt the ramekin so that the sugar covers all the custard.

Arroz con Leche

Cal 240
VEGETARIAN

Difficulty: Normal
Preparation time: 20 minutes
Cook time: Well over 5 hours
Servings: 4

Nutrition per serving (g)

Fat	Saturates	Carbs	Sugars	Protein
3	2	47	20	10

Ingredients

- 6 quarts water (and more as needed)
- 1, 12 oz can evaporated milk
- 1 cup brown rice
- 3 cups water
- 4 teaspoons maple syrup
- ¼ teaspoon ground cinnamon
- ½ teaspoon vanilla extract
- ¼ cup raisins

Method

1. Pour the water into a pot and get it to simmer.
2. Once simmering, place an unopened can of evaporated milk in the water.
3. Let simmer for 5 hours. Keep checking the water levels. The water must always be covering the can.
4. Remove the can from the water and let cool completely.
5. Place 3 cups of water on to boil then add the brown rice.
6. Reduce the heat to a simmer and let the rice cook for about 40 minutes or until the water has evaporated. If the water evaporates and the rice has not finished cooking, keep adding a little water at a time until the rice is done.
7. Add the evaporated milk, maple syrup, cinnamon, and vanilla extract to the rice.

8. Stir thoroughly and let simmer for 20 minutes. Stir periodically throughout the cooking to make sure everything is incorporated and it isn't getting caught on the bottom of the pan.

9. Add the raisins and cook for a further 5 minutes. At this point, the pudding should be thick and creamy in consistency. If not cook for a bit longer so that more of the liquid can evaporate.

10. If you want the rice to be softer, just keep adding a little bit of water and continue cooking.

11. Once you are happy with the rice and the consistency of the pudding, switch off the stove and take it off the heat.

12. Allow it to cool completely before placing it in the fridge for at least an hour.

13. Serve on its own or with some fresh fruit on top.

Flan

Cal 125

VEGETARIAN
GLUTEN-FREE

Difficulty: Normal
Preparation time: 20 minutes
Cook time: 35 minutes
Servings: 6

Nutrition per serving (g)

Fat	Saturates	Carbs	Sugars	Protein
3	1	17	12	6

Ingredients

- ¼ cup granulated sugar
- ½ cup water
- 1, 4 oz carton egg substitute
- 2 large egg yolks
- ¼ cup granulated sugar
- 1 tablespoon pure vanilla extract
- 2 cups 1% milk
- 2 quarts water

Method

1. Place a saucepan on the heat. Add the sugar and water in it and heat it up.
2. Allow it to boil until it changes to a brown color. If it changes color unevenly, swirl the pan.
3. Once the caramel is done, pour equal amounts into 6 ramekins.
4. Preheat the oven to 325 degrees Fahrenheit.
5. Get out a bowl and pour in the egg substitute, egg yolks, sugar, and vanilla extract. Mix until combined.
6. Boil some water in a kettle or on the stove.
7. Pour some milk into a clean saucepan and place it on the stove to heat.
8. Keep stirring it. Once it starts to boil, remove from the heat.
9. Slowly pour the milk over the egg mixture and whisk continuously.
10. Once it has all been combined, pour into the ramekins.

11. Place the ramekins in a roasting dish and fill it with the boiling water. The water should come halfway up the ramekin.

12. Place in the oven to cook for 35 minutes.

13. Once cooked, remove from the oven and water bath.

14. Leave to cool.

15. Once cooled place plastic wrap over the top of them and leave in the fridge for at least 4 hours.

16. When you are ready to serve them, run a knife around the sides to loosen the flan.

17. Turn over onto a plate and serve. If it does not come out immediately, tap the top of the ramekin.

Sweet Potato Tarts

Cal 119
VEGETARIAN

Difficulty: Normal
Preparation time: 20 minutes
Cook time: 100 minutes
Servings: 12

Nutrition per serving (g)

Fat	Saturates	Carbs	Sugars	Protein
2	0	22	4	2

Ingredients

- 4 quarts water
- 20 oz sweet potato, cubed
- 4 oz ginger snaps
- 1 tablespoon maple syrup
- ¾ cup 2% milk
- ½ teaspoon ground nutmeg
- 2 tablespoons of sugar
- 2 teaspoon vanilla extract
- ⅛ teaspoon salt
- 2 large eggs (separated)

Method

1. Preheat the oven to 325 degrees Fahrenheit.
2. Place a pot of water on the stove to heat up.
3. Once the water is boiling add the sweet potatoes. Let boil for 40 minutes, until soft.
4. Once cooked, drain and place on a plate with paper towels.
5. While the potatoes are cooking, place the ginger snaps in a food processor. Process until they turn into crumbs.
6. Pulse and drizzle in the syrup.
7. Get out a muffin tin and line with cupcake liners.
8. Pour the ginger snap mixture into each liner. Pat it down so the bottom is fully coated.
9. Place it in the oven and let it cook for about 10 minutes. Remove and set aside to cool.

10. Take the cooked and cooled potatoes and mash them. They should be a smooth consistency.

11. Mix in the milk, nutmeg, sugar, vanilla extract, salt, and egg yolks. Set aside.

12. Whisk the egg whites until they form stiff peaks.

13. Fold the egg whites into the sweet potato mixture. Do not overmix.

14. Distribute the batter into the muffin tins.

15. Place in the oven and let it bake for 40 minutes.

16. Remove from the oven when cooked through and leave to cool before serving.

Papaya, Yogurt and Walnut Boat

Cal 184

VEGETARIAN

Difficulty: Easy
Preparation time: 5 minutes
Cook time: 0 minutes
Servings: 2

Nutrition per serving (g)

Fat	Saturates	Carbs	Sugars	Protein
9	1	21	15	9

Ingredients

- 1 medium papaya, halved
- ½ cup plain fat-free or low-fat Greek yogurt
- ¼ cup walnuts
- ¼ teaspoon ground cinnamon

Method

1. Use a spoon to scoop out all the seeds from the papaya.
2. Fill the halves with yogurt and then top with the walnuts.
3. Sprinkle the cinnamon on top and serve.
4. You can easily eat this dish with a spoon. Try and get everything in one bite.

Conclusion

Now that you have come to the end of the book, you have the knowledge you need to create an acid reflux friendly lifestyle. Not only do you have lots of delicious recipes to try, but you also have the necessary knowledge every person that suffers from acid reflux needs to have. Hopefully, you have already tried some of the recipes and have discovered that being on an acid reflux diet does not mean that you have to compromise flavor and diversity in your meals. There are so many amazing recipes to try, so I'm sure you won't run out of things to cook anytime soon.

As you get more accustomed to using the ingredients that are acid reflux safe, it will become like second nature. You don't have to stick to these recipes rigidly. Feel free to modify, add, or take away ingredients to create new flavors and new dishes. Eventually, you will find your style and the flavors you love.

I hope the information in this book has given you the inspiration and the knowledge to kick off a better lifestyle. Keep learning and trying new recipes. This journey does not have to be boring or repetitive. I know that this is just the first step to a healthier and happier life.

Others books by Robert Dickens

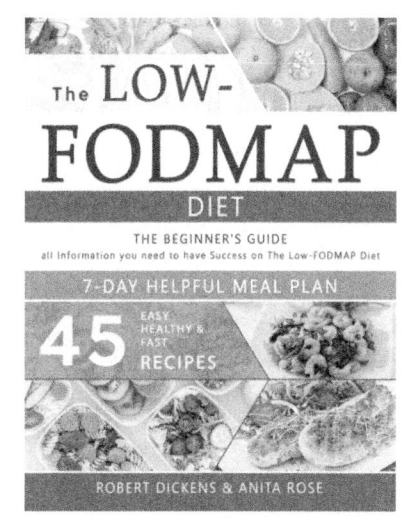

The Low-FODMAP diet

The Beginner's Guide, including 7 days Meal Plan + 45 Easy, healthy & fast recipes and all information you need to have Success on The Low-FODMAP Diet

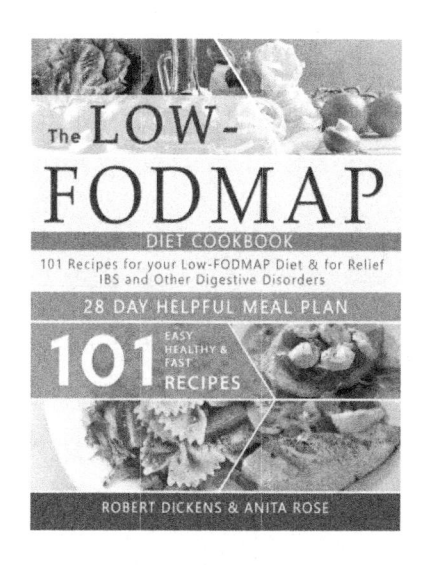

Low FODMAP diet cookbook

101 Easy, healthy & fast recipes for yours low-FODMAP diet + 28 days helpful meal plans

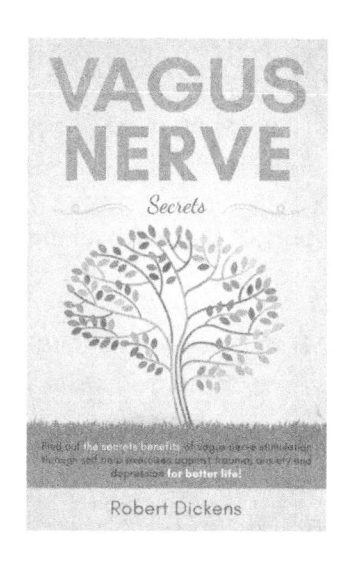

Vagus nerve secrets

Find out the secrets benefits of vagus nerve stimulation through self help exercises against trauma, anxiety and depression for better life!

References

Brohl, P. (2020, March 2). *7 Smoothies for Acid Reflux (and GERD).* Vibrant Happy Healthy. https://vibranthappyhealthy.com/smoothies-for-acid-reflux

Chirichigno, J. (2018, December 7). *Simple Food Swaps for 8 Heartburn Triggers.* One Medical. https://www.onemedical.com/blog/get-well/heartburn-trigger-replacements

Cunha, J. P. (2017, October 25). *GERD (gastroesophageal reflux disease) FAQs - frequently asked* questions. RxList. https://www.rxlist.com/quiz_gerd_gastroesophageal_reflux_disease/faq.htm

Davenport, T. (2018, November 6). *Acid reflux: Meal plan for a week.* Health Central. https://www.healthcentral.com/article/reflux-free-meal-plan-for-a-week

Dr. Gourmet. (n.d.). *Free GERD / acid-reflux friendly recipes that are easy and healthy from dr. gourmet.* https://www.drgourmet.com/gerd/index.shtml

Gotter, A. (2015, March 23). *What to Drink for Acid Reflux.* Healthline. https://www.healthline.com/health/gerd/beverages#smoothies

MacGill, M. (2017, November 13). *Acid reflux: Causes, treatment, and symptoms.* Www.Medicalnewstoday.Com. https://www.medicalnewstoday.com/articles/146619

Madell, R. (2020, January 28). *7 Foods to Add to Your Diet for Acid Reflux.* Healthline. https://www.healthline.com/health/gerd/diet-nutrition#foods-to-avoid

McClees, H. (2020, June 30). *Food Swaps That Can Provide Acid Reflux Relief.* One Green Planet. https://www.onegreenplanet.org/natural-health/food-swaps-that-can-provide-acid-reflux-relief/

RefluxMD. (n.d.). *Recipes For People With Acid Reflux.* RefluxMD. https://www.refluxmd.com/acid-reflux-recipes/

SelectHealth. (n.d.). *6 natural remedies for heartburn.* SelectHealth. https://selecthealth.org/blog/2017/09/6-natural-remedies-for-heartburn

Verywell Fit. (n.d.). Heartburn-Friendly Recipes. Verywell Fit. https://www.verywellfit.com/heartburn-recipes-4157043

WebMD. (2002, February 6). *Complications of Heartburn and GERD.* WebMD; WebMD. https://www.webmd.com/heartburn-gerd/guide/untreated-heartburn#1

All images have been sourced from www.unsplash.com - www.freepik.com

© **Copyright 2020 - All rights reserved.**

The content contained within this book may not be reproduced, duplicated or transmitted without direct written permission from the author or the publisher.

Under no circumstances will any blame or legal responsibility be held against the publisher, or author, for any damages, reparation, or monetary loss due to the information contained within this book, either directly or indirectly.

Legal Notice:
This book is copyright protected. It is only for personal use. You cannot amend, distribute, sell, use, quote or paraphrase any part, or the content within this book, without the consent of the author or publisher.

Disclaimer Notice:
Please note the information contained within this document is for educational and entertainment purposes only. All effort has been executed to present accurate, up to date, reliable, complete information. No warranties of any kind are declared or implied. Readers acknowledge that the author is not engaged in the rendering of legal, financial, medical or professional advice. The content within this book has been derived from various sources. Please consult a licensed professional before attempting any techniques outlined in this book.

By reading this document, the reader agrees that under no circumstances is the author responsible for any losses, direct or indirect, that are incurred as a result of the use of the information contained within this document, including, but not limited to, errors, omissions, or inaccuracies.

Printed in Great Britain
by Amazon